DISASTER
PREPAREDNESS
AND
MANAGEMENT

D0223769

DISASTER
PREPAREDNESS
AND
MANAGEMENT

Michael Beach, DNP, ACNP-BC, PNP

Assistant Professor
University of Pittsburgh School of Nursing
Pittsburgh, Pennsylvania

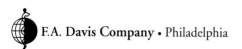

F.A. Davis Company • Philadelphia

F. A. Davis Company
1915 Arch Street
Philadelphia, PA 19103
www.fadavis.com

Printed in China

Last digit indicates print number: 10 9 8 7 6 5 4 3 2 1

Publisher, Nursing: Joanne Patzek DaCunha, RN, MSN
Director of Content Development: Darlene D. Pedersen
Project Editor: Christina C. Burns
Art and Design Manager: Carolyn O'Brien

As new scientific information becomes available through basic and clinical research, recommended treatments and drug therapies undergo changes. The author(s) and publisher have
done everything possible to make this book accurate, up to date, and in accord with accepted
standards at the time of publication. The author(s), editors, and publisher are not responsible
for errors or omissions or for consequences from application of the book, and make no war-
ranty, expressed or implied, in regard to the contents of the book. Any practice described in
this book should be applied by the reader in accordance with professional standards of care
used in regard to the unique circumstances that may apply in each situation. The reader is
advised always to check product information (package inserts) for changes and new information regarding dose and contraindications before administering any drug. Caution is especially urged when using new or infrequently ordered drugs.

Library of Congress Cataloging-in-Publication Data

Beach Michael, 1952-
   Disaster preparedness and management / Michael Beach.
      p. ; cm.
Includes bibliographical references and index.
ISBN-13: 978-0-8036-2174-9
ISBN-10: 0-8036-2174-4
1. Disaster nursing. 2. Emergency management. I. Title.
[DNLM: 1. Disaster Planning—methods. 2. Disaster Planning—organization & adminis-
tration. 3. Disease Outbreaks—prevention & control. 4. Terrorism—prevention & control.
WA 295 B365d 2011]
RT108.B43 2011
610.73'49—dc22
                                                                                     2009052690

This book is dedicated to my wife for her love, patience, kindness, understanding, and wisdom that she has shown not just through this project but throughout our 33+ years of marriage. Without her, this would not have been written and I would not be who I am.

Reviewers

Susan D. Clayton, MSN, RN

Instructor
Barton College
Wilson, North Carolina

Maureen Cluskey, PhD, RN, CNE

Associate Chairperson Department of Nursing
Bradley University
Peoria, Illinois

Valerie Cochran, MSN, RN, NE-BC

Assistant State Nursing Director
Alabama Department of Public Health
Montgomery, Alabama

Denise Danna, DNS, RN, NEA-BC, FACHE

Assistant Professor, Associate Dean
Louisiana State University Health Sciences Center School
    of Nursing
New Orleans, Louisiana

Corinne C. Fessenden, PhD, RN

Associate Professor
Blessing-Rieman College of Nursing
Quincy, Illinois

Michelle Ficca, RN, PhD

Associate Professor and Graduate Coordinator
Bloomsburg University
Bloomsburg, Pennsylvania

L. Sue Gabriel, MSN, MFS, EdD, RN, SANE-A, CFN

Associate Professor
BryanLGH College of Health Sciences, School of
   Nursing
Lincoln, Nebraska

Linda Grimsley, RN, DSN

Associate Professor & Chair, Department of Nursing
Albany State University
Albany, Georgia

Beverley Holland, PhD, ARNP

Associate Professor of Nursing, BSN Department Chair
Bellarmine University, Lansing School of Nursing and
   Health Sciences
Louisville, Kentucky

Marilyn K. Rhodes, EdD, MSN, RN, CNM

Colonel (retired), USAF, NC
Assistant Professor
Auburn University at Montgomery
Montgomery, Alabama

Donald G. Smith Jr., BSN, MA, PhD, RN, ACRN

Assistant Professor
Hunter School of Nursing, Hunter College
City University of New York
New York, New York

Janice S. Smith, RN, PhD

Associate Professor
Shenandoah University
Winchester, Virginia

Laura Terriquez-Kasey, RN, MS, CEN DMAT Nurse

Assistant Clinical Professor
Decker School of Nursing
Binghamton University
Binghamton, New York

Acknowledgments

Thanks to David Karpinski, Jim Ressler, and Jane Cambest for their help involving the research required for this text. Thanks also to Joanne DaCunha, Christina Burns, and Jen Schmidt from F.A. Davis for their prodding and patience on this project (I am sure I did not show my gratitude at the time). Lastly, thanks to my family for their patience and understanding for all the family events I missed or cut short because "I was working on the book."

Contents

Introduction

What This Book Is and What It Is Not

If you are looking for a book that will give you all the answers to all the questions concerning disaster preparedness and response, look no further because it simply does not exist. It cannot exist. Such a book would require volumes of information and more importantly, knowledge of the future. Disasters, by their very definition, overwhelm all available resources. As such they will overwhelm any disaster preparations. They are fluid events that cannot be predicted. We cannot know what effect our preparations will have. We cannot stop the inevitable. Lives will be disrupted, injuries and death will occur, property will be damaged, public services and health care will not be able to provide the standard of care normally expected by the public. If the scope of the disaster is large enough, these things are simply unavoidable. No book can encompass everything we need to know to avoid the unavoidable. If this scares you, that is understandable. But, don't let it paralyze you.

What this book attempts to do is provide the basic information you need to ask the right questions, so that you can find the answers that will minimize the effects of disasters and mass casualty incidents. In this book are chapters dealing with the basics of disaster, personal preparedness and awareness, hospital preparedness, triage, weapons of mass destruction, violence, and other pertinent topics. It provides a relatively in-depth explanation of these topics so you, the practicing nurse, nurse practitioner, other advanced practice nurse, student, or other health-care professional can apply the information to your practice. From the information in this book, you should be able to understand how your practice will change in a disaster or a mass casualty incident. You should develop a sense of what you need to be aware of concerning rare diseases, many of which begin very much like a simple case of the flu or other common diseases. You should be able to form questions concerning your level of preparedness and that of the institution you work for. These questions will then guide you into forming a plan to minimize the devastating effects of disasters. They will help you to be as prepared as possible.

I suppose the question should be asked, if we are going to be overwhelmed, why should we even try? The answer lies beyond the concern about regulations, certifications, and the like. The answer is simple. We are responsible because of our practice and to those we care for—by virtue of what we do and who we are—to be as prepared as possible. We simply must try. We owe it to our patients/clients/colleagues/friends/family, both ethically and morally, as an extension of our daily responsibilities to them.

We owe it to our employees. As administrators, we have the obligation to care for our employees and to enable them to do their jobs to the fullest extent possible. During a disaster or mass casualty incident, it will be difficult physically, emotionally, and professionally for nursing and other health-care professionals to perform their duties. We need to provide the tools that enable them to function as best as possible in this austere environment. We can do this through education by encouraging undergraduate programs to include disaster education as part of their curriculums. We can provide continuing education to our employees on a regular basis so that they have the information they need to respond when an event occurs. We can provide a plan, the supplies, and equipment to carry out the tasks that will be so desperately needed in a disaster.

We owe it to ourselves. By being able to care for ourselves and minimize the effects of a disaster as much as possible, we stand a better chance of surviving the event and it is okay to want to survive. By being prepared, we are less the victim we might have been. It is imperative that we can care for ourselves by preparing responsibly for whatever risks we believe may affect us. Personal preparedness provides us with a level of comfort during those very austere times. Being aware and alert to both the dangers and the good in life will help us live a fuller, more meaningful life. We prepare for the bad and enjoy the good.

So how should you use this book? Use this book to develop a basic understanding of the topics covered. Use this book to inspire you to find other information through other books, online sources, and articles. Use this book to think critically and apply the information to your practice. Use this book to develop research questions and work with others to find the answers to those questions. Use this book to begin to find the evidence, or if it is not there, develop the evidence needed to guide our practice. Most importantly, use this book to ask questions that only you can answer; that will make you, your institution, your school, and your family better able to withstand those impending disasters. We know disasters are coming, at least we think they are coming. We are not sure when or what, but by answering those questions, we will be better prepared for the possible, inevitable disaster.

Disaster Basics

Introduction to Disaster Basics

A disaster can be defined in several ways, but in all cases it is a destructive event that overwhelms all available resources. A disaster may originate as natural or manmade and may be intentional or accidental. Within the hospital setting, they may be internal or external. A natural disaster is caused by the forces of nature such as a hurricane, tornado, or earthquake. A manmade disaster may be the result of a terrorist act or industrial accident. In this case, the terrorist act would also be intentional whereas the industrial accident would be accidental. Within the hospital setting, internal disasters are those that affect the structure or effectiveness of the hospital; for example, disruption of essential utilities or physical damage threatening the structural integrity of the building. External disasters are caused by disruption and damage outside the hospital. External disasters may cause disruption within the hospital and also cause large numbers of victims, which may overwhelm the hospital. In all cases, disasters overwhelm all available resources. Depending on the scope of the disaster, the available resources may be local, state, federal, or multinational.

During the past 100 years, disaster response (DR) has changed significantly. Events during the late 1800s and early 1900s caused tremendous levels of destruction and loss of human life, amplified by a lack of organized preparation and response. In 1906, San Francisco, California, was rocked by a major earthquake. Rescue efforts were carried out primarily by victims with limited organized help from local officials and public servants such as law enforcement and fire fighters.

Much of the city burned owing to a lack of trained response personnel and water. Evacuations were unorganized and ineffective. There was no plan for moving victims to safety; rescue began spontaneously by the victims themselves. Victims who were trapped were rescued by other victims as fire fighters fought the fires.[1]

In 1889, a wall of water 60-feet high rushed over Johnstown, Pennsylvania, killing 2209 people. Blame was placed on unregulated changes made to an earthen dam situated above the city and the estimated 10 inches of rain that fell in the previous 24 hours. Many victims died trapped in the wall of debris that collected against a railroad trestle and burned for days. Calls went out for morticians and coffin makers. Donations for recovery were received from as far away as Europe. The only official organization that was able to respond was the recently formed American Red Cross.[2] Today, each of those locations would be declared a disaster area by its governor and there would be an intense federal response in the form of trained personnel, equipment, and money. A massive influx of aid for a structured organized response would engulf the areas.

As disaster response has become more formalized, disaster planning has taken on increasing importance. Authorities at all levels of government and institutions are mandated to both prepare for unanticipated disasters and to take steps to both prevent disasters from occurring. They must take steps to lessen the impact of all types of disasters.[3,4] Phases of disaster preparation and response have been defined. Mitigation and preparation are actions taken before the event to lessen the effect of a disaster. Response is the activity during and immediately following a disaster with the intention of rescuing victims and saving property. Recovery is the slow process of rebuilding and returning to normal life and, lastly, evaluation and the applications of lessons learned concerning the effectiveness of past preparations and response, which may make future preparation and response more effective and mitigate the effects of the next disaster.[5,6]

An in-depth understanding of the disaster cycle, the incident command system, and other points discussed in this chapter is important to nursing and other health-care professionals from four perspectives—education, practice, administration, and research. It is essential that nurses be educated about disasters, the preparations that are taken for them and why they are taken, the recovery effort, and application of lessons learned from the past for application in future events. A well-educated nurse and advanced practice nurse become valuable resources within the health-care community for both preparation and response. That education begins with an understanding of the basics as a student.

For nursing and advanced practice nursing practice, this information helps to define roles in disaster planning and response. Past events have shown that management decisions during disasters and as preparations are made concern both knowledge and authority. Authority without knowledge may not lead to optimal outcomes. Nursing and advanced nursing practice, with an adequate understanding of disasters and preparations, become a valuable resource.

Nursing administration affects the largest professional workforce and, therefore, the largest response unit in any health-care institution. Effective knowledge of the phases of the disaster cycle provides a clear understanding of the importance of mitigating the potential for disasters. It also helps administrators realize the importance of a well-educated and prepared nursing and advanced nursing workforce. There is often good understanding of disease and trauma processes, which will be discussed in later chapters; however, there are other areas in which anecdotal evidence is the only evidence guiding practice. Nursing researchers should work to establish a deeper understanding of disaster preparation and response.

Phases of Disaster Response

The Disaster Cycle is made up of four phases—mitigation, response, recovery, and a return to mitigation of future disasters. It is not possible to designate any of the phases as first. Mitigation in both instances involves an analysis of what has worked or failed in the past, what improvements in technology have been developed, the changes in demographics and populations, and changes to infrastructure. How well an individual, hospital or government responds and the extent of the disruption caused by the event are directly dependent on effective preparation. This makes the mitigation portion of the cycle very significant. The cycle is continuous. Each phase has its own restrictions and necessities. **See Figure 1–1.**

Mitigation comprises the preparations taken to lessen the effects of a disaster. Mitigation may take the form of physical improvements, such as infrastructure improvements, stockpiles of food and water, or organizational preplanning. **Response** is the organized or unorganized action taken during and immediately after the event. Its purpose is to save life, limb, and property. Response is carried out in an unorganized manner by the victims themselves, called *self-rescue*, or in an organized manner as in the case of local, state, or federal disaster response personnel. **Recovery** is the effort to return to normalcy after a disaster. It is usually a long, difficult process. Recovery is complicated by several factors including finances and personal freedoms. The cycle then

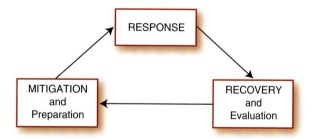

FIGURE 1–1. The Disaster Continuum. Mitigation lessens the effects of a potential disaster with preplanning. Response to an event depends on preplanning. Recovery is the long process of returning to normal day-to-day life and may take years. Through the recovery phase, evaluation of past efforts and subsequent lessons learned help to prepare more effectively for the next disaster, bring the process back to mitigation.

continues. Lessons learned from the event and an analysis of the effectiveness of preparations and response help to mitigate the next event.[7]

Mitigation

Mitigation is any planning and preparations taken to minimize the effects of manmade or natural disasters. It may take several forms. The levies built along rivers to control flooding or storm basements for shelter during tornadoes are examples of mitigation. Building codes requiring buildings to meet certain standards that reduce the chance of fire and contamination and improve structural safety are another. In earthquake-prone areas, these codes require that structures meet standards that will minimize damage and danger during an earthquake. Stockpiling food, water, medicine, and other supplies is another form of mitigation and preparation. Stockpiling may be as simple as individuals or families developing a personal preparedness plan or as complex as development of the federal government's stockpiles of medications, vaccines, food, water, and other supplies for large disaster response.

Mitigation also takes the form of organizational efforts and planning. Organizing in anticipation of what may occur is essential to mitigating the effects of disasters. Hospitals, schools, other institutions, and governments should develop organizational charts showing who has authority and knowledge to respond; assigning areas of responsibly to prepare for and respond to a disaster. These organizational charts become very complex, but they allow roles of individuals within the hospital or other setting to be delineated and they establish clear lines of authority. Organization allows individuals, families, institutions, and governments to mount an orderly and effective response to any event even as it overwhelms the available resources.

An important aspect of mitigation is risk assessment. The risk assessment identifies what events the individual, community, state, or nation is at risk for. For example, the western coast of the United States is at risk for earthquakes whereas the Gulf Coast is not. The Gulf Coast is at risk for hurricanes whereas the Ohio Valley may only feel the remnants; however, these remnants may cause flooding. Severe weather is a concern for most parts of the United States, though the specific type will differ. Industrial areas may be at risk for chemical spills or releases, or fires. Transportation routes regularly carry hazardous materials. All areas of the world may be at risk for pandemic emergencies. Each type of disaster requires somewhat different planning and response, and many health care certifying organizations, such as The Joint Commission, now require an all-hazards approach to disaster planning. Institutions must plan and be able to respond to not only individual risks but also whatever event may present.[6]

The risk assessment must be realistic. Large metropolitan areas may be at risk for terrorist attacks and institutions located there may need to take measures to care for large numbers of victims. Smaller towns and institutions may mistakenly believe that they are not at risk for terrorism and thus feel no need to prepare for more than a few victims beyond day-to-day operations. Large numbers of victims may present either from a local disaster or terrorist attack or as overflow from nearby areas. Individuals and families should conduct their own risk assessment. There may be risks associated with everyone in one area whereas events such as flooding may affect only a few. It is important to realize that institutions that may have provided help in the past, may be affected by the same problems and concerns as an individual or family in the event of a disaster. Properly done, the risk assessment will point out what may happen, how the emergency systems can respond, and what steps need to be taken to make that response most effective. Risk assessment allows those with responsibility, be it personal responsibility or responsibility for the nation, to decide what should be mitigated and how.[6]

An example of this is the changes made after the attacks on the United States on September 11, 2001. Since these attacks, air marshals regularly fly both domestic and international flights as undercover security and airport security has been increased. After subsequent attempts to smuggle explosives onto airplanes as liquids, security was increased again. Liquids are now restricted to very small amounts and are inspected separately. Attempts to smuggle a shoe bomb have now necessitated passengers' shoes to be removed and examined separately during the security screening. Careful attention should be placed on the risk assessment. It is impossible to predict or prepare for every eventuality, but plans should be developed that facilitate an effective response to any disaster.

Response Phase

The response phase is the mobilization of forces during and immediately after an event to save life, limb, and property. It is both an organized response by trained personnel and a grassroots effort by victims who may be able to help themselves and those around them. Its effectiveness is dictated by the scope of the event and preparations made during the mitigation phase. Response is first performed by victims and trained rescue personnel within and close by the event. Trained rescue personnel and untrained volunteers from nearby areas not severely affected by the event will respond next. Finally, state and/or federal rescue personnel will respond after requests to the state's governor or the federal government.[6]

Professional Response Personnel

Professional response personnel are limited to a relatively small group of trained professionals organized locally or on a state or federal level who may be mobilized to respond to a disaster. There may be volunteers, who in every way embody the standards of professional disaster response, but because of issues within the response system, they may or may not be able to respond as professional responders. On a federal level, these professionals include:

- Disaster Medical Assistance Teams (DMAT).
- Disaster Mortuary Operational Response Teams (DMORT).
- Veterinary Medical Assistance Teams (VMAT).
- Search and Rescue teams (SAR), each part of Homeland Security through the Federal Emergency Response Agency (FEMA).

- Each branch of the military has teams specifically trained to respond to terrorist attacks and other incidents, such as radiological or biological emergencies.
- Federal Law Enforcement Agencies (LE) have units dedicated to respond to terrorist attacks.
- The Centers for Disease Control and Prevention (CDC) has personnel who can respond to disease outbreaks for support and advice.
- The military may respond as it did during Hurricane Katrina, providing rescue for stranded victims, and medical aid.
- The United States Public Health Service Commissioned Corps also responds to public health emergencies related to disasters.
- The National Guard responds to disasters through orders from the state's governor providing aid and security.[6]

On the local level, health-care professionals include:

- Physicians.
- Advanced practice nurses.
- Nurses.
- Emergency service personnel and other professionals.

Each of these groups falls under different sources of authority and will respond based on differing levels of requests. The National Guard responds under orders from the state's governor at the request of local authorities. The governor also may ask the federal government for assistance if the scope of the disaster goes beyond what can be handled by local and state resources. FEMA can then respond providing extensive medical, mortuarial, veterinary, and SAR personnel and resources. DMAT hospitals can be set up to supplement local hospitals and to provide clinics in remote areas. SAR personnel can assist in finding and transporting victims. Morticians assist in victim identification and veterinarians provide care for domesticated and wild animals. Other requests to the federal government may bring the Coast Guard or other military personnel to supplement medical, SAR, and transportation needs. Each of these groups is trained for the rigors, both physically and mentally, of disaster response. They are familiar with and part of the Incident Command System discussed later.[6]

Local health-care providers respond as part of the organized local response. Hospitals and clinics provide for the needs of victims by expanding their normal operations. They team with outside aid to meet the needs of those affected by the disaster.

Other agencies also are capable of providing needed aid during a disaster, such as the Red Cross, Red Crescent, or the Salvation Army. These groups are made up of a mix of volunteers and paid personnel. They provide food, water, and other needs including shelters for those displaced. These are well-organized national groups with a very organized deployment and support structure ensuring that they do not place an additional burden on local authorities.

The Incident Command System

The response to any disaster, small or large, should be as organized as possible. To facilitate this, the Incident Command System (ICS) should be initiated as soon as an event is anticipated. The ICS allows for a strong, definitive command structure with specific areas of responsibility assigned to individuals as needed and is applicable to the community's response as well as that of hospitals and other institutions. It is designed so that there is one incident commander (IC) with centralized authority over the operation. Directly under the IC there may be additional command staff, as needed, which is made up of an assistant, media relations officer, and safety officer, each with specific duties and under direct command of the IC. In addition, the IC overseas operations, planning, logistics, and finance designed to meet the needs of the response. Each of these areas is under the direct control of an individual who answers to the IC. More areas may be added if needed, but most should fall under one of the established areas of control. The system is designed so that there are three to five individuals directly under the control of any one leader. As groups tasked under a specific control group become larger than five or so people, they are broken up into two groups, each under its own leader answerable to the head of that section. If the number of groups grows larger than three to five, then leaders are designated to control only three to five or so of the groups[6] **(see Fig. 1–2).**

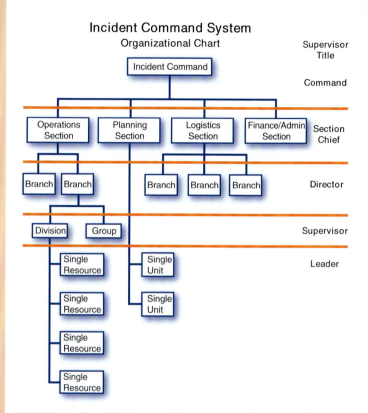

Incident Command System
Organizational Chart

Supervisor Title

Incident Command — Command

Operations Section | Planning Section | Logistics Section | Finance/Admin Section — Section Chief

Branch | Branch | Branch | Branch | Branch — Director

Division | Group — Supervisor

Single Resource | Single Unit — Leader

Single Resource | Single Unit

Single Resource

Single Resource

FIGURE 1–2. The Incident Command System is an organized command structure that allows for only three to five people under any one person's direct control. It expands and contracts to fit the scale of the event.

The **Operations** section is concerned with carrying out the tasks necessary for the disaster response. They would include groups such as law enforcement, fire, SAR, medical, and any other field operations. If there are three law enforcement teams, they would become their own subset under operations. The same would apply to the fire service, medical, or SAR. The leaders of each team would answer to a leader for the subsection. These leaders would answer to the operations chief. **Logistics** concerns itself with transportation, supplies, equipment, and base operations. Its task is to obtain, organize, and maintain supplies and equipment, organize and maintain base operations, and provide for transportation needs. **Finance** tracks all expenditures including money, man-hours, or supplies. Finance is an integral aspect of the event response. Tracking costs, man-hours, and supplies used in the response is essential for budgetary concerns and the possibility that there may be reimbursement after the event.[6]

If multiple agencies respond to an event, such as federal agencies, the military working with state and local response, or if multiple aspects of the same service come together, such as multiple law enforcement groups, the system is designed to allow the command structure to expand. Sub-commanders representing each group work with the IC advising him or her of their capabilities and facilitating communication with their individual groups. This change is a product of the National Incident Management System (NIMS). NIMS was developed when it was found that communication would break down as multiple agencies came together, that centralized command was in jeopardy, and to facilitate leadership from those with the most knowledge and experience. NIMS allows each group to contribute its specialized service while allowing for a centralized command structure. Communication is facilitated as each group is allowed to use its own system. Each area retains command of its section but is assigned by the IC to perform specific tasks allowing for expertise in each area. All participants are aware of and are working toward the central goals of the operation.[6]

The ICS is designed to expand and contract as necessary and to adapt to the needs of the institution and incident. At its smallest, it only needs an IC controlling one group; at its largest there would be one IC with several leaders from other organizations and multiple groups under each section. If the event encompasses a large enough area, smaller, local incident command centers or posts may be established, each controlling its territory and answering to the IC. These also may expand and contract as necessary. Hospitals may use the ICS as a command structure within their institution in the event of a disaster. The hospital ICS designates a command and function structure based on established authority lines and functions within the hospital.[6] Operational units would function within the units of the hospital. Specialty units may be designated to perform triage, patient transportation, and other patient care functions. Other logistical units would provide supplies and other needs throughout the hospital. The IC would provide overall direction while the section leaders and those under them would provide functional leadership for the operations of the hospital or clinic.

Recovery Phase

The **recovery phase** begins after the response phase ends. More realistically, the response phase fades out as the recovery phase fades in. The recovery phase is the slow return to normal life after a disaster. Although normal life may not be the same as it was before the disaster, life has changed from the intense efforts to save life, limb, and property. During this time, victims will begin to move from shelters back to their homes or into temporary housing. Permanent housing will be re-established. Utilities will begin to be restored and food, water, fuel, and other necessities will be available, though possibly not at predisaster levels. Schools, business, and local government will slowly begin to function again. Many aspects of life taken for granted before the disaster may have changed or may have disappeared entirely.

The health-care system; municipal services including the fire service, law enforcement, the courts; and EMS should be priorities. Each is essential to the care of people as they return. Disasters may destroy essential structures and equipment for hospitals, municipalities, EMS, and the fire service. All may have lost personnel; they will certainly be overwhelmed. Returning each of these to functional status should be a priority. State and federal resources and personnel may assist until local resources are functional again.[6]

Completing the disaster cycle is the transition from the recovery phase into evaluation and preparation for the next event. Evaluation of the preparations for and response to the disaster is essential to mitigate the effects of the next disaster.

Throughout recovery, individuals, families, businesses, and authorities have come to realizations concerning how they could have prepared better or what should have been done differently during response. These lessons learned and changes made in future planning and preparations bring the disaster cycle full circle, back to mitigation.[6]

Nursing and Health-Care Implications

Health-care institutions and individuals are required by legislation and certifying bodies to be prepared and to respond to disasters. Beyond these concerns, health-care providers have an ethical duty as an extension of the everyday care provided to the public to be prepared to care for victims of disasters.[8–11] Physicians, hospital administrators, and emergency services have increased their level of preparation for disaster planning.[4,5,12–14] Competencies have been established for health-care providers that suggest extensive education involving all aspects of disaster planning and disaster response.[9,15,16] Nursing also has established competencies that address concerns such as chain of command, the role of nursing in disaster planning and disaster response, communication concerns, and addressing knowledge deficits.[15] Programs also are being developed to meet the specific needs of advanced practice nurses and nurse practitioners.

Of note is the Columbia University Bioterrorism Curriculum Development Committee's report that established four competency areas for health-care providers. The Columbia University Bioterrorism Curriculum Development Committee was established in 2003. Educators from nursing, medicine, public health, and other aspects of health-care education examined the necessity of disaster education for health-care providers and established core competencies for both students and clinicians. The four areas include:

1. Emergency Management and Preparedness including:
   - Understanding of disaster phases
   - Understanding of Risk Assessment and Planning

- Roles within disaster planning and disaster response
- Understanding the Incident Command System and National Incident Management System
- Integration with community disaster planning and disaster response
- Examination of communication concerns
- Knowledge of available resources
- Understanding of planning evaluation, including drills and exercises

2. Terrorism and Public Health Preparedness including:

- Knowledge of Chemical, Biological, Radiological, Nuclear, and Explosive (CBRNE) agents

3. Public Health Surveillance and Response including:

- Understanding and applying the principles of surveillance for public health emergencies and disasters
- Understanding and applying public health interventions

4. Patient Care including:

- The ability to perform histories and physicals, develop differential diagnosis, order diagnostics, evaluate and treat victims of disaster-related events
- Understand the need for and perform forensic evaluations

The first three competencies are meant to be part of every health-care educational program whereas the last is a clinician competency that applies to all clinicians, particularly nurse practitioners, physician assistants, and physicians[9] **(see Table 1–1).**

The implications are that health-care providers must be well educated and well prepared to respond to disasters that overwhelm all available resources. The roles of health-care providers are not easily defined in a disaster; all personnel must be educated and prepared to respond in whatever manner they are called upon.

TABLE 1–1 Columbia University Core Competencies for Health-Care Providers Concerning Disaster Education and Response

Student competency 1: Emergency Management and Preparedness including:

- Understanding of disaster phases
- Understanding of Risk Assessment and Planning
- Roles within disaster planning and disaster response
- Understanding the Incident Command System and National Incident Management System
- Integration with community disaster planning and disaster response
- Examination of communication concerns
- Knowledge of available resources
- Understanding of planning evaluation, including drills and exercises

Student competency 2: Terrorism and Public Health Preparedness including:

- Knowledge of Chemical, Biological, Radiological, Nuclear, and Explosive (CBRNE) agents

Student competency 3: Public Health Surveillance and Response including:

- Understanding and applying the principles of surveillance for public health emergencies and disasters
- Understanding and applying public health interventions

Clinician competency 4: Patient Care including:

- The ability to perform histories and physicals, develop differential diagnosis, order diagnostics, evaluate and treat victims of disaster-related events
- Understand the need for and perform forensic evaluations

The core competencies established by Columbia University for all health-care providers. Competencies 1, 2, and 3 are general and intended for health-care students; competency 4 is intended for practicing clinicians.

Summary

Disasters are destructive events that cause death, injury, or property damage and disrupt normal life to such a degree that they completely overwhelm all available resources and the ability to respond. They may be natural or man-made, accidental or intentional, internal or external; the distinctions may overlap.

The disaster cycle is an ongoing process that begins with mitigation and preparation during which we learn from past experiences and prepare so that we may respond to future disasters more effectively. It is performing a risk assessment that identifies potentially hazardous events that may affect the community or institution. The mitigation phase continues as planning and preparations are made to lessen the deleterious effects of the disaster. The response phase immediately follows the disaster and utilizes all of the preparations that have been made. It is the organized and unorganized efforts to decrease loss of life and limb and damage to property. The authority structure that enables an organized and safe response is the Incident Command System part of the National Incident Management System. The recovery phase is the slow process of rebuilding and returning to normal life. It involves reassessing the risks and effects of the disaster and evaluation that allows us the opportunity to learn from the disaster and decide what reasonably can be done to lessen the negative effects in the future. Each action and decision should encompass what has been learned from the event, its response, and from past disasters to mitigate the effects of the next one.

Nursing and other health-care groups should provide an in-depth understanding of disasters and disaster preparation within their respective educational programs. Students should graduate with the ability to understand what has been done to prepare in the past, the effectiveness of those preparations, and what should be done to lessen the effects from future events. This education and continued education of the workforce will help to define the roles nursing, medicine, and other members of the health-care team will take to effectively manage disaster preparation and response. These roles include management, section leaders, triage, treatment, transportation, and other functions that may or may not have fallen to nursing in the past. Nursing and advanced practice nursing should expect to use all of their skills and education in ways beyond normal day-to-day operations.

Nursing research is needed to examine the effectiveness of disaster education for the nursing workforce, the roles nursing has played in past events and how nursing, advanced practice and registered nurses, can be utilized optimally in the future to care for overwhelming events.

SUGGESTED INDEPENDENT STUDY COURSES

The following are Suggested Independent Study Courses available through FEMA and the Department of Homeland Security.

Federal Emergency Management Agency, Independent Study, Course Name: *Introduction to Incident Command System, 1-10.* Course Code: IS-100.a, accessed at http://training.fema.gov/IS/crslist.asp

Federal Emergency Management Agency, Independent Study, Course Name: *Introduction to the Incident Command System for Healthcare/Hospitals.* Course Code: IS-100.HC, accessed at http://training.fema.gov/IS/crslist.asp

Federal Emergency Management Agency, Independent Study, Course Name: *Introduction to the Incident Command System, I-100, for Law Enforcement,* Course Code: IS-100.LEa, accessed at http://training.fema.gov/IS/crslist.asp

Federal Emergency Management Agency, Independent Study, Course Name: *Applying ICS to Healthcare Organizations,* Course Code: IS-200.HC, accessed at http://training.fema.gov/IS/crslist.asp

Federal Emergency Management Agency, Independent Study, Course Name: *Disaster Basics,* Course Code: IS-292, accessed at http://training.fema.gov/IS/crslist.asp

Federal Emergency Management Agency, Independent Study, Course Name: *Community Hurricane Preparedness,* Course Code: IS-324, accessed at http://training.fema.gov/IS/crslist.asp

Federal Emergency Management Agency, Independent Study, Course Name: *National Response Framework, An Introduction,* Course Code: IS-800.b, accessed at http://training.fema.gov/IS/crslist.asp

REFERENCES

1. U.S. Geological Service. Earthquake hazards program. Available at: http://earthquake.usgs.gov/regional/nca/1906/18april/index.php. Accessed March 14, 2007.

2. National Park Service. Johnstown flood national memorial. Available at: http://www.nps.gov/archive/jofl/home.htm. Accessed March 14, 2007.

3. Bureau of National Disasters. Mitigation emerges as major strategy for reducing losses caused by natural disasters. *Science*, 1999;284(18).

4. Waeckerle JM, Seamans S, Whiteside M, White S, Murray R, on behalf of the Task Force of Health Care and Emergency Services Professionals on Preparedness for Nuclear, Biological and Chemical (NCB) Incidents. Executive Summary: Developing objectives, content, and competencies for the training of emergency medical technicians, emergency physicians, emergency nurses to care for casualties resulting from NCB incidents. *Annals of Emergency Medicine*. 2001;37(6): 587–601.

5. Hogan DM, ed. *Disaster Medicine*. 3 ed. Philadelphia, PA: Lippincott; 2007.

6. Department of Homeland Security, ed. National Incident Management System. Washington, DC: 2008;156.

7. Veenema TG, ed. *Disaster Nursing and Emergency Preparedness*. 2 ed. New York, NY: Springer; 2007:656.

8. Kane-Urrabazo C. Duty in a time of disaster: a concept analysis. *Nursing Forum*. 2007;42(2):56–64.

9. Markenson DM, DiMaggio C, Redlener I. Preparing health profession's students for terrorism, disaster, and public health emergencies: core competencies. *Academic Medicine*. 2005;80(6):517–526.

10. Farmer JC, Carlton PK Jr. Hospital disaster medical response: aligning everyday requirements with emergency casualty care. *World Hospitals & Health Services*. 2005;41(2):21–24.

11. Kgalegi P, Chetty M. Disaster preparedness. *World Hospitals & Health Services*. 2007;43(1):17–22.

12. Alexander AJM, Glen W, Mazurik L. A multiphase disaster training exercise for emergency medicine residents: opportunity knocks. *Academic Emergency Medicine*. 2005;12(5):403–411.

13. Rottman SJMF Shoaf, K, Dorian, A. Development of a training curriculum for public health preparedness. *Journal of Public Health Management Practice*. 2005;November (suppl):S128–S131.

14. Westphal RMM, Jewell S, Skawinski, E. Development of an online bioterrorism preparedness course. *Journal of Public Health Management Practice.* 2005;November (Suppl):S132–S134.

15. Tichy MM, Bonds E, Beckstrand R, Heise B. NP's Perceptions of disaster preparedness education: quantitative survey research. *American Journal For Nurse Practitioners.* 2009;13(1):10–22.

16. Hsu EB, et al. Healthcare worker competencies for disaster training. *BMC Medical Education.* 2006;6:19.

Triage

Introduction to Disaster Triage

What follows is an adaptation of a somewhat popular ethical question.

You are standing next to an incapacitated person on a railroad track. There is an oncoming train. You have very limited resources. You may or may not be able to save this person from the oncoming train. There also are other tracks and other incapacitated people whom you may or may not be able to save from the trains hurtling down the tracks toward them. Can you walk away from that one person knowing that possibly some of the others may be saved using your limited resources? You know that by walking away this person will probably die. You know that her care would take an extremely large portion of your limited resources, but she may live; she may have functional deficits, but others may live if you go to them, or they may not. The point is that they need you; would you walk away to help somebody else who has a better chance of survival? **(See Fig. 2–1.)**

Disaster triage asks you to do just that. To face the possibility of walking away from one person in favor of treating others who have a better chance of survival; to use the available resources to treat the maximum number of patients who have the best chance of survival.[1-3] In this chapter, we will discuss how triage is used on a day-to-day basis in emergency departments (ED) and other aspects of health care. We will examine how triage is used in hospitals during a disaster or mass casualty incident (MCI) and we will examine the use of triage in the field, outside of the hospital setting during these same events.

Nursing will be called upon in practice to perform triage of victims from disasters and mass casualty events. During the initial triage, they will move quickly to decide who is both sickest as well as who can be saved. In a disaster, those who cannot be saved may be victims who under other circumstances would receive significant resources in the form of supplies and time. Nurses must be prepared to make those decisions. In subsequent triage, secondary triage, and more, the nurse will be called upon to decide who is treated first, who goes to radiology, and what initial treatments can be done under the circumstances. Nurses may then need to decide on and administer treatment without the safety net of practitioners and physicians. Advanced practice nurses may be ideally suited to triage. They have an understanding of both medicine and nursing. With additional

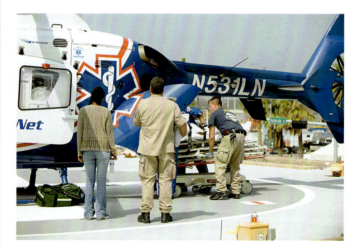

FIGURE 2–1. Galveston Island, Texas, September 19, 2008. Members of the disaster medical assistance team (DMAT) and medical flight crew put a patient into a helicopter for transport to an area hospital. The DMAT is set up at the University of Texas Medical Branch as a mobile emergency site following the disruption of power and services to the area caused by hurricane Ike. Triage in the field provides patient sorting, initial treatment, and then arranges transportation to the most appropriate hospital. *Photo by Jocelyn Augustino/FEMA.*

knowledge and training, they would be equipped to make rapid decisions concerning patient care. An understanding of this process should be a part of undergraduate education, continuing education, and through hospitals and professional societies.

Triage is a French word meaning to sort. Triage was first used by a surgeon in Napoleon's army. The process of triaging separates patients or victims based on the severity of their illness or injury.[3] During a disaster, it is the process of deciding who is to be treated first, who can wait, and whose life cannot be saved.[1,3–5] During the day-to-day functioning of EDs, it is the process of deciding who needs to be brought in immediately for treatment and who can wait. Triage is used daily in EDs, intensive care units, and in many other aspects of health care. On a national scale, we, in effect, triage health insurance eligibility. Those who can afford to pay for health insurance or have it as a benefit from their employer, have health insurance. The elderly are eligible for Medicare. For those who are left, we as a nation have decided that the remaining limited resources will provide health insurance, through Medicaid, only for the poorest of children and the disabled without other sources of coverage. Anyone who does not fit into these categories is not covered. At this writing, we have decided that we, as a nation, cannot provide health insurance for everybody with our limited available resources. In the ED and disaster settings, we triage patients according to the patient's or victim's severity of illness or trauma. In the ED, we have the available resources to attempt to save all patients regardless of condition. Except under a very few circumstances, all patients presenting to the ED who are acutely ill or severely injured will be seen and treated faster and all available resources expended on them.[4,6–8] By triaging or sorting patients based on the severity of illness or injury, we are able to identify and treat those patients who will die unless they are seen immediately. We are able to identify those patients with minor concerns and those who may deteriorate quickly. In an environment where patients are often asked to wait for significant amounts of time for treatment, this information is essential. In a disaster, available resources are overwhelmed and we can only try to save those victims with a good chance for survival.

During a disaster or MCI, it is essential to quickly decide who is stable, who needs to be treated as quickly as possible, and who will be given comfort measures but are not expected to survive. Triage during a normal day in the hospital setting may take several minutes or longer, during a disaster or MCI it must be performed in less than 1 minute. Triage during a disaster evaluates a few critical signs: is the victim breathing, do they have a pulse, can they follow commands. Vital signs are not taken and little consideration is given to the specifics of the victim's injury. We only want to know if they are stable, if they can be saved under the circumstances, and how long can they wait for treatment. Triage, under these circumstances, categorizes victims according to those few basic considerations that indicate if the victim can survive and in what order they should be treated. This is essential in a disaster or MCI when there are not enough resources to treat every victim with the same standard of care we use under normal circumstances. Some victims may not be seen for days, the most severe may wait hours, and those who cannot be saved, will be allowed to die.

Disasters completely overwhelm all available resources. Similarly, MCIs stretch available resources but do not overwhelm them.[8] Patients, who under daily circumstances would utilize large amounts of time, personnel, and materials regardless of their chance of survival, may receive only comfort measures in a disaster. Those with minor injuries will wait, possibly significant periods of time, before being treated while those who can be saved are treated first.[1,2] Hospital triage will concentrate on efficient use of radiology suites, ultrasound examinations, computed tomography (CT) scanners, and operating rooms while in the field, responders will be deciding who needs to go to which hospital first and how they will get there.[4] Triage is one of the most difficult, ethically and professionally challenging tasks in any environment and is made significantly more so in disaster settings[1,3,4,9–11] (see Fig. 2–2).

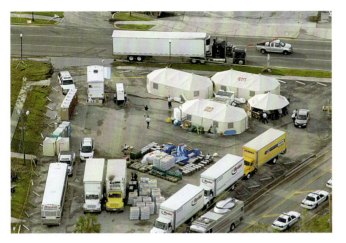

FIGURE 2–2. Punta Gorda, Florida, August 16, 2004. Aerial image of disaster medical assistance team (DMAT) tents in front of the hospital in Punta Gorda. DMATs were operational the day after hurricane Charley. Tents such as these provided by the DMAT may be used to triage patients at the hospital and ease patient flow. *FEMA Photo by Andrea Boohe.*

Patient or Victim Triage Classifications

Patients triaged during normal daily hospital functioning, are classified according to the severity of their illness or injury, in other words, according to their acuity. Patients with a higher acuity, that is, more severe illness or injury are treated with a higher priority. They are treated first, and a larger degree of resources, such as time, money, supplies, pharmaceuticals, and manpower, are spent on them. Patients with a lower acuity may wait until others are treated before they are fully cared for. Patients may be classified according to a three-tiered, emergent, urgent, nonurgent classification or a five-tiered system. The five-tiered system consists of Level 1, Emergent; Level 2, Urgent; Level 3, Acute; Level 4, Routine; and Level 5. These classifications may be applied under any day-to-day circumstance, either in the field by emergency medical services (EMS) or in the hospital setting by nurses, physicians, and practitioners. During a disaster or MCI, triage must be performed quickly with little available information.

A color-coded disaster tag system allows for quick recognition of the patient's acuity level and is generally red/immediate, yellow/delayed, green/minor, and black/deceased or expectant. They are numbered for identification when there is no victim's name and have other benefits during a disaster or MCI. Both systems are used to identify the level of acuity of the patient or victim; some tag systems may even use the emergent, urgent, nonurgent terminology, but there are significant advantages to the color-coded tag system during a disaster or MCI. Both types will be discussed.

The Emergent/Urgent/Nonurgent Patient Classification and the Emergency Severity Index

By assessing the patient's level of acuity, the most severely ill or injured are treated first and those with minor concerns treated last. One triage system used in hospital settings on a day-to-day basis utilizes the emergent, urgent, and nonurgent classifications, with emergent being the highest patient acuity and nonurgent being the lowest.[12,13] They may be described as follows:

- **Emergent.** Any seriously injured or acutely ill patient is classified as Emergent. This would include significant or potentially significant trauma from a motor vehicle crash, fall, or industrial accident in which there is the possibility of death or disability-causing injury. Acutely ill individuals, especially children and the elderly, are also considered emergent. This may include chest pain and severe abdominal pain, respiratory distress from a variety of causes, and certain headaches or neurological issues. Respiratory or cardiac arrests and other instances in which the patient is dying, also are considered emergent. These patients are taken immediately into the ED for treatment. Hazardous material exposure should also be considered emergent, particularly for children.

- **Urgent.** Patients classified as Urgent are those who need to be treated as quickly as possible, but do not have a life-threatening illness or injuries. They are stable. This would include some abdominal pains; some headaches; known trauma without threat to life, limb, or disability; respiratory and head, ears, eyes, nose, and throat (HEENT) illnesses; or other system illnesses and other concerns. These patients should be reassessed often for worsening of their condition.

- **Nonurgent.** The Nonurgent classification is reserved for those with minor injuries or illnesses such as suture removal and minor wounds.

Besides this system, there is a five-tiered Emergency Severity Index system that helps to differentiate patients on the extreme ends of the scale. Emergent patients are divided into those who require immediate care and those who will deteriorate rapidly if they are not treated. Nonurgent patients are further categorized into those with chronic or routine complaints and those who will require no utilization of resources. The system is described next:

- **The Emergency Severity Index**
  - Level 1—Emergent
    - Patients require immediate care without which they will die; they are immediately seen and treated. Examples include cardiac or respiratory arrest, severe bleeding, unresponsive patients, or those in shock.
  - Level 2—Urgent
    - These patients should be seen quickly by a physician or practitioner because of the potential for rapid deterioration. Examples include patients with active chest pain, signs of stroke, or high-risk patients with high fever.
  - Level 3—Acute
    - These patients are acutely ill with symptoms that may indicate serious illness, but are not in danger of rapid deterioration. Examples include abdominal pain, nausea, and vomiting.
  - Level 4—Routine
    - These are patients with chronic and routine complaints without threat to loss of life, limb, or eye sight. Examples

include simple urinary tract infections, lacerations, or sprained ankles or knees.
- Level 5
  - These are patients who are stable and will require no testing for treatment.

A significant difference between day-to-day triage and disaster or MCI triage is the care provided to those victims who either are dying or are expected to die. In the day-to-day triage (when the Emergent/Urgent/Nonurgent Classifications or Emergency Severity Index is used) a significant amount of time and resources are generally expended to resuscitate and treat patients who may or may not have a positive outcome or may survive for a short time. In a disaster, victims who probably will not survive are classified as "expectant." In this instance, "expectant" refers to someone who is, unfortunately, expected to die. This classification may occur during initial or secondary triage.[1,3,4,10,11,14]

Color-Coded Classification System (Tagging)

Triage in an MCI or disaster event incorporates a classification system different from the Emergent/Urgent/Nonurgent System or Emergency Severity Index.[14] Color-coded triage tags with green/minor, yellow/delayed, red/immediate, and black/deceased or Expectant are used to identify the victims and the seriousness of their injuries. There are several types of triage tags available for use. All are similar.

The ideal tag should be:

- Color-coded to indicate the victims' acuity level.
- Numbered so that a definite identifier is attached to each victim.
- Large enough for documentation of important information.
- Able to attach to the victim, not their clothing **(see Fig. 2–3).**

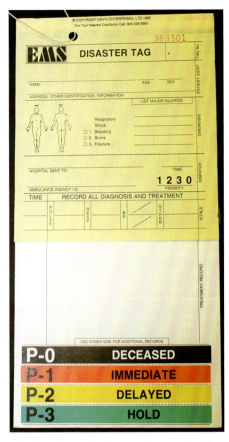

FIGURE 2–3. This is a picture of a disaster triage tag. The disaster tag should be clearly color-coded with detachable color tabs at the end of the tag, be easily attachable to the victim, and have adequate space for essential documentation. *Photo by Nam H. Do.*

The colors and their meaning are as follows:

- **Green/Minor:** These victims have minor injuries. They are often termed the "walking wounded" because they are able to follow commands **and** walk to a collection point. They will wait the longest for treatment.

- **Yellow/Delayed:** These victims may not be able to walk, but they are stable and will be transported or treated after seriously injured victims, those tagged Red or Immediate, are cared for.
- **Red/Immediate:** These victims are seriously injured and show signs of being unstable. These victims will be treated and transported before any other victim.
- **Black/Expectant/Deceased:** These victims are deceased or are expected to perish without significant use of resources, which are either not available or more appropriately used on others. Comfort measures are provided for the victim.

The color coding tag is arranged so that green is the outermost color with yellow next, followed by red, and then black. Each color is a perforated tab so that it may be removed starting with green as the outer most and black as the closest to the body of the tag. If the condition is green nothing is removed. For yellow, the green is removed and so on to the removal of red for a victim tagged as black if they are an expectant or deceased victim. Victims who were previously classified as minor or delayed may deteriorate and become immediate or red and someone classified as immediate may become expectant or deceased; however, victims should never be triaged backward, that is they should not go from a red or immediate to yellow or delayed. Victims may appear to be stabilizing only to worsen quickly.[3–5,14,15] This is particularly true of children. Once the decision is made concerning a victim's level of acuity, he or she should remain

WHY IS IT IMPORTANT To Never Triage Backward?

Never triage backward. Victims may deteriorate and become either more of a priority or become expectant and receive comfort measures only, but they should never be seen as getting better. Whatever caused the triage officer to classify someone at a certain level should remain. Secondary triage should only decide who of the immediate victims should be treated or transferred first and if any of the victims have now deteriorated. Victims classified as delayed may become immediate, but they should never become minor.

either at that level or one that is more severe if they begin to deteriorate **(see Table 2–1).**

Tags should be clearly numbered with an area to document the victim's identifiers. If possible, a duplicate tag with the same number should be available to be attached to any of the victim's belongings. Belongings may be removed from the victim in some instances, but should travel with the victim.[14] For instance, a victim who requires decontamination. All of the victim's clothes, jewelry, wallet, and other personal belongings would be placed in a plastic bag and tagged with the same number as the victim.

Tags should have space for documenting vital signs, treatment, or other comments and the time they were performed. This may be the only record of a victim's condition and treatment until a traditional chart is established. The tag should become part of the victim's record and may

TABLE 2–1	Color Coding of Disaster Tags	
COLOR	STATUS	CONDITION
Black	Expectant or deceased	Victims deceased or not expected to recover under the austere circumstances with limited resources.
Red	Immediate	Victims with the most severe injuries or illnesses who will benefit most from the limited resources in the austere environment. Those severely injured or ill who are expected to recover.
Yellow	Delayed	Victims with potentially serious injuries or illnesses but who are able to wait until those more in need are transported or treated.
Green	Minor	Victims who are "the walking wounded." They are injured but are able to wait until the victims designated as immediate or delayed are transported or treated.

provide vital information affecting the care of the victim. This area should be waterproof, allowing information to be written while wet. The area will be small by necessity; comments will need to be concise and accurate.[5,14] Documentation is critical throughout the triage process. It is also extremely difficult. Although there may be a traditional chart eventually, each victim's tag should contain all pertinent patient information. This tag travels with the victim and carries that information to subsequent caregivers. Any procedures and medications, vitals and their times are recorded. Under dire and austere circumstances, this documentation may be all that is possible and available for long periods of time.[3]

Two things are essential concerning tags. First, all of the EMS, Emergency Response personnel, and hospitals in the local area should use the same tags. In a crisis situation, everyone should be familiar with the same system. Second, *use the tags*. In a crisis, the emphasis is often on speed and this is important, but it is essential to be familiar with and follow the appropriate steps to avoid negative outcomes. Not properly identifying and tracking victims leads to confusion over identity, victim condition, and treatment history, and concerns from next of kin.[2,14]

There has been research into improvements for the color-coded tagging system. Computerized models used to triage and track victims throughout the process are being developed.[5,16]

WHY IS IT IMPORTANT To Include Documentation on the Triage Tags?

Document clearly and concisely on the triage tag; it may be the only significant record of victims' care and status as they move from the incident to the hospital or morgue. This has significant implications in judging the status of the victim, if they are deteriorating, and what has been done to stabilize the victim to determine what has worked or may not have. This documentation may also have legal implications and provide information to help identify those who are unknown.

Although there may seem to be a correlation between the three classification systems discussed, the process of assessing and assigning the victims in a disaster or MCI is extremely different. The Emergent/Urgent/Nonurgent System and Emergency Severity Index classifications use a more thorough assessment and require a deeper understanding of the patient's condition, whereas the disaster/MCI system requires an extremely rapid assessment and only a limited understanding of the patient's injuries or illness. In the field, during a disaster or MCI, the color-coded system would certainly be used. At the hospital, under the same circumstances, the same color-coded system would be used initially, but secondary triage would incorporate more advanced assessment skills and knowledge.

Everyday Triage Versus Disaster Triage in the Hospital Setting

Triage in the Everyday Hospital Setting

Daily triage in the hospital setting primarily takes place in the ED, but aspects of the process are used throughout the hospital. Patients with minor injuries or illnesses may have to wait to be seen until after those who are acutely ill or injured are treated. When a patient presents who is severely injured or in cardiac or respiratory distress or arrest, they are treated immediately. In short, the sicker or more severely injured a patient is, the faster he or she will be cared for and with more resources.

Deciding who is more acutely ill is not always obvious. A headache may be a simple tension or migraine headache or it could be a subdural hematoma. Abdominal pains could be simple gastritis or may be peritonitis from an acute appendicitis. These complex decisions should be made by an experienced, well-educated registered nurse who is well trained in the triage protocols established at the hospital. Careful, clear, concise questions should provide most of the information needed to distinguish acute illnesses from minor concerns. A careful but focused and brief physical examination including a complete set of vital signs is also necessary. Any patient who needs to wait before being seen in the ED should be retriaged every 15 minutes and as necessary. Any change in condition should be noted and the order in which patients are brought in for definitive treatment, may change (**see Table 2–2**).

TABLE 2–2 Types of Triage	
HOSPITAL DAY-TO-DAY TRIAGE	**HOSPITAL MCI OR DISASTER TRIAGE**
Emergent: Those patients with potentially life-threatening illness or trauma or trauma that may potentially be life threatening.	**Immediate:** Those victims who are seriously injured or ill who have the best chance of survival under the circumstances. There may be other victims who are more seriously injured or ill but do not have a good chance of survival.
Urgent: Those patients with potentially serious illnesses but are stable and may wait until after the emergent patients are treated.	**Delayed:** Those victims who are seriously injured but whose injuries or illness, at the moment, is not life threatening. They are breathing, perfusing, and following commands within acceptable parameters under the circumstances.
Nonurgent: Those patients with minor illnesses or concerns that may wait until emergent and urgent patients are seen.	**Minor:** The "Walking Wounded," these victims may be injured or ill, but are stable with only very minor wounds that may be treated hours or days later.
Deceased: Only those patients who are deceased. Patients who are emergent but have DNR (do not resuscitate) orders are treated as emergent until the orders are confirmed.	**Deceased or expectant:** Those victims who are deceased or who are injured so badly or are so acutely ill that they cannot be saved with the limited resources.

When an MCI, such as a large bus accident with many injured children or a large industrial accident, occurs that does not overwhelm the resources within the community or ED, the priorities and structures of triage change. With an MCI, more victims than the hospital normally cares for present from the incident and will need to be triaged, tagged, and treated. In addition to these patients, the hospital's regular patient population will also present as usual. The local resources, while not overwhelmed, are stretched. Additional physicians, practitioners, nurses, and other personnel may be called in from off duty or other parts of the hospital to supplement the normal daily staff.[2,4,5,8,17] Protocols allowing nurses to order basic radiological studies or laboratory tests and initiate treatment protocols may expedite patient treatment.[18,19] One note of caution, patients sent for radiological studies should be prioritized so that the most critical are cared for first. Although this may be obvious, what may not be obvious is that as additional victims from the MCI arrive, there may be critical patients needing immediate testing. CT scans and standard radiological studies should be reserved for head, chest, and abdominal studies. Most stable obvious fractures and sprains should not be sent to radiology until the incident has resolved. Immediate treatment should include splinting and evaluation for and, if necessary, restoring distal neurovascular function and comfort measures, including pain control; radiological studies should be delayed.

Triage and tagging in the hospital setting during an MCI ensures that critical patients from the incident and the acutely ill regular population are seen first. Those less critical may have to wait before being seen. Resources may be stretched and additional personnel may be called in, but the system is not overwhelmed.[3,4,18,19] All patients are seen and treated in a timely manner according to normal standards of care. Priorities do change allowing for radiological suites, ultrasound, CT scanners, and operating rooms to be held open for critical victims presenting from the incident. Patients who do need to wait must be reevaluated regularly for changes in condition and priority. All patients are identified and though disaster tags may be used, normal patient tracking and charting may be in effect.

During a disaster, triage in the hospital setting incorporates some of the structures of MCI triage with some significant differences. In both situations, potentially large waves of victims will present to be triaged and tagged; however, in the disaster setting, resources are not just stretched, they are overwhelmed. There are not enough personnel, supplies, equipment, or space to treat the number of victims.[1,4,5,8,10,19] While triage personnel in the field will tag and send only critical victims to the ED, many victims will self transport, and Good Samaritans will transport other victims to the hospital who may or may not be critical. Providers in this setting will need to decide who has minor injuries or concerns that need to wait, perhaps a very long time, for treatment, and may only be seen and treated by nurses.[18] The hospital triage personnel will need to decide which of the critical patients will be treated first and what limited testing may be carried out.[1,2,4,10,18,19] More difficult are the decisions concerning which patients will receive comfort measures only and be allowed to die.[1,11] Separate holding areas should be established for each group of victims. Personnel should be assigned to each area to continuously retriage the victims and administer comfort measures as needed.

Assuming that they are functional, radiological suites, ultrasound services, CT scanners, and operating rooms should be used only for the most critically ill or injured victims. After the needs of the critical are met, those with lesser injuries may be tested or sent to surgery. Supplies also will be limited. Oral fluids, antibiotics, pain and other medication should be considered for each patient instead of IV fluids and medications.[10]

Victims should be organized according to their level of acuity; according to how they are tagged. All victims tagged as minor should be assigned a holding area where they can be monitored for a short time after which they may be sent home with instructions to return later. Victims tagged as

WHY IS IT IMPORTANT To Reserve Resources During an MCI or Disaster?

During an MCI or disaster, it is essential to reserve the operating suites and radiology cares, particularly the CT scanners, for the most severe patients. If radiological studies will help determine treatment, for instance to rule in or out internal injuries, traumatic brain injuries, or other concerns that may require surgery, then they become priorities. The operating suites should be reserved for those procedures that will save life or limb. Even during a lull in the number of victims presenting to the hospital, significant consideration should be made before sending routine cases to either radiology or the OR. Victims often present in waves and a lull may only be the calm before the storm. Routine treatment and testing, such as obvious fractures, should wait.

delayed will require closer monitoring and will remain at the hospital until treatment. These holding areas will require personnel to monitor and care for victims. Victims tagged immediate should be treated as soon as space and personnel are available. Victims expected to succumb to their injuries should have a separate holding area with personnel available to provide comfort measures as needed. Lastly a larger temporary morgue may need to be set up to hold the deceased.

It is critical that a triage officer be assigned early in the process and limit his or her activities to organizing and directing all matters concerning triage. Although she may direct the administration of some medications or procedures in the victim holding areas, her main function is to classify patients and direct what order patients are treated or sent for preliminary testing. She should be a practitioner or physician with significant patient care experience. She needs to remain calm within a confused, intense environment. Decisions will need to be made quickly, decisively, and with little remorse. She will need to be compassionate and communicate both this compassion and her decisions clearly. It is likely that this will be the most difficult position within the disaster response.[1,3,4]

The size of the disaster and number of patients will dictate how many nurses and other personnel such as social workers or admissions personnel are placed under the triage officer.[4] If the holding areas for minor, delayed, critical, and expectant patients are separated by distance or structure, then an officer, responsible to the triage officer, should be assigned to each of these areas. Teams of paramedics or nurses in combination with practitioners or physicians may be necessary if large numbers of victims present all at once or in rapid succession. This team approach also may be necessary at the location of a large MCI or at designated treatment locations in the event of very large-scale disasters. Paramedics or nurses on the team should act with a large degree of autonomy with the practitioner or physician supervising and organizing the team (see Table 2–3).

Nurses providing care, administering medications, and reevaluating victims should be assigned to treatment or holding areas as needed. Social workers should be assigned

TABLE 2–3 The Roles of Hospital Personnel in the Triage Area During a Major MCI or Disaster	
Physicians	Triage officer, triage and patient/victim treatment
Practitioners and physician assistants	Triage officer, triage and patient/victim treatment
Registered nurses	Triage and patient/victim treatment, patient/victim histories
Paramedics	Triage and patient/victim treatment, patient/victim histories
Social workers	Patient/victim identification, comfort, family liaison
Nurses aides	Patient/victim transport, monitoring, comfort, patient/victim identification, and history
Admissions personnel	Patient/victim identification, family liaison, comfort
Volunteers	Patient/victim transport, monitoring of noncritical patients/victims, comfort

to provide comfort and care within their abilities. Admissions personnel should be assigned to assist with victim identification and tracking. Care should be taken in assigning these personnel. They should be well trained in the disaster response process and the realities of patient care in austere environments. This will be difficult both physically and psychologically. Patient care under these conditions would not be the normal day-to-day standard of care.[1,3,4,8,10,17] All personnel must understand that these conditions may require care to be directed by a nurse instead of a practitioner or physician or that "comfort measures only" may be provided to those patients who would normally be treated with all available resources, but who now are expected to expire. Actions that under the normal standard of care would be negligence or criminal may be necessary and appropriate during a disaster response.[1,11]

Triage in the Field During an MCI or Disaster

Triage in the field, at the scene of the MCI or at designated treatment areas during a disaster, becomes necessary when there are more victims than the available EMS personnel can quickly extricate, provide initial care, and transport to the appropriate treatment facility. This trigger point will be different for each community. In large metropolitan areas, or where several towns are close together, each with their own services, there may be several ambulances and personnel to respond allowing for several victims to be cared for and transported quickly. In more rural areas there may only be one or two ambulances, few emergency medical technicians (EMTs) or paramedics, and few first responders who can respond to an incident.[20] In this instance, a multivehicle crash may cause many more victims than can be handled quickly and some victims would need to wait while more critical victims are transported first. Deciding who is treated first, who will wait, and possibly who may only receive comfort measures is the responsibility of the field triage officer.[1,3,11,21]

In the event of an MCI or disaster, the most experienced paramedic or EMT on the scene should be designated as the triage officer; however, the first EMS personnel to arrive should immediately begin to triage the victims. The triage officer is the person who organizes and manages the victim collection and directs both the care of the victims and their transport to one, or perhaps many treatment facilities. This is a daunting task and several decisions need to be made quickly.[1,4]

If the event is large enough and there is a significant number of victims, a victim collection area should be established. Those victims, for whom it is appropriate, should be moved to this area for monitoring, treatment, and to await transport to a treatment facility. The designated victim treatment or collecting areas should be large enough to hold the number of expected victims. In a large-scale disaster, victims will present to these treatment areas in waves. Just as they would to the hospital, they will present on their own, and be brought in by Good Samaritans and rescue personnel. Ideally, an area with controlled access on two sides is the best choice. All victims should be funneled to an entry area where they are triaged, identified, tagged, and brought to the appropriate treatment or holding area. There should be a separate exit area. The exit should allow for ambulances and other transportation to maneuver in and out of the area. Priority victims, those tagged immediately should be nearest this exit.

Weather is a significant concern when choosing the victim collection area. Rain or snow, as well as bright sun, and hot or cold temperatures will require shelter. Heaters may be necessary in the winter whereas fans or air conditioning may be necessary in the summer for long-term operations. Rain and snow will turn open, unpaved ground into mud or slush. This will affect both motorized and walking traffic. Under disaster circumstances, the victim collection area may need to be functional for a long time and much consideration is needed in deciding its location. An MCI also may require victims to remain in the area for a few or perhaps several hours. Even a few hours exposed to the elements will have deleterious effects on a victim.

Communication

Communication during the triage process is challenging and complex. The triage officer at the scene or his or her designates needs to be aware of and may be called upon to communicate the following:

- Number of victims in each category and the number and classification of victims found but still in the field
- Where they are and who should be rescued first
- Number of ambulances and where they are going
- The general condition of the most critical victims

The triage officer at the hospital needs to be aware of and may need to communicate the following:

- Number of victims presenting to their facility
- Number of victims the facility is prepared to care for
- Number of victims in each category
- Who is to be sent to radiology, the operating room, or treatment areas first
- How many ambulances are in route and the condition of the victims they are transporting

This requires a clear and constant flow of information.[2–4,17,21]

Unnecessary communication should be avoided. For example, the field triage officer should inform the hospital triage officer when they are sending victims. The victim's identifiers, such as triage tag number, the condition, and estimated time of arrival should all be included. The ambulance crew should not communicate with either the hospital or the field triage area unless absolutely necessary or requested by the hospital or field triage officer. If information is relayed through the radio operator or through another station or unit because of distance or other concerns, the person relaying the information should repeat the information completely, using the same words as the original message if possible. Communication in the confused circumstances of an MCI or the austere and confused atmosphere of a disaster is very challenging.

WHY IS IT IMPORTANT To Have Clear and Concise Communication?

Communication should be clear and concise and be limited to that from Triage Officer in the field to the Triage Officer at the hospital. During a disaster, there is a lot of information that needs to be communicated. Anxiety and stress will affect everyone involved. Because of this, communication becomes very difficult. Before speaking into a phone or radio, take a moment to decide what needs to be said and how to say it. Avoid speaking too quickly, using jargon or clichés, or providing personal information that is unnecessary. Always remember that others may be listening, more importantly, the information you are providing may save a person's life.

Victim Triage

Triage in a very broad sense is the organizational process described; however, **victim triage,** the actual assigning of victims to the appropriate level of acuity is the heart of the triage process. Victim triage is the assessment and evaluation of each victim, assigning each to a particular level of acuity and attaching the disaster tag with the appropriate color exposed. Although assigning officers, organization, and establishing the victim collection area and other tasks are extremely important, they should not substantially delay victim triage in either a disaster or MCI. It is essential to begin to triage the victims and then to begin to treat and transport those in most need and who will benefit the most by this care. This process has just that as its primary goal: to identify those victims who will benefit the most from the limited available resources.[1,3]

There are few differences between triage in an MCI and that of a disaster other than the scope of the incident and victim collection. MCIs are often contained within a relatively confined area. Those victims who are able to move will self-extricate to the periphery of the incident and seek assistance. Those not able to self-extricate can be found within the immediate area of the incident. Depending on the magnitude of the MCI, this may be a large area requiring an organized

WHY IS IT IMPORTANT   To Have Rapid and Efficient Triage?

Triage at the event should be rapid and efficient, taking no more than 60 seconds per victim. Triage at the hospital also may use this method if faced with huge waves of victims. Treatment should be limited to very few life-saving measures such as opening the airway or attempting to control significant bleeding. Secondary triage then takes a somewhat closer and timely assessment of the victims. During secondary triage, decisions are made concerning who is transported and where they will be sent. Further treatment of injuries may also be completed during secondary triage.

search and rescue operation. In a disaster, the defined area of the incident is much larger. Again, those who can self-extricate may seek assistance or they will begin to assist themselves and others; others, due to the scope of the disaster, will remain where they are and wait for help. It will almost certainly require search and rescue to find some of the victims.[4]

All victims, either when found or when they present for aid, must be evaluated quickly and efficiently. As discussed, they need to be classified as minor, delayed, immediate, or expectant/deceased. No significant treatment is given by the person performing triage, instead they classify the victim according to a few significant parameters while others follow and treat those who have already been triaged.[3] Those victims who are mobile, and those able to be moved after evaluation, should be moved to a designated collection area. Those who cannot be moved or who are in need of more complex extrication also should be classified and their location marked for extrication and further care.

The person performing triage should not stop to treat the victim beyond lifesaving measures and only those who may be done quickly, such as opening the victim's airway or a pressure dressing applied over major bleeding.[3] If these measures fail or cannot be accomplished in 60 seconds or less, the triage person should tag the victim as expectant/deceased and move on to the next victim. It is the responsibility of the personnel who follow to provide care to the victims as prioritized by the triage officer or person. When all of the victims have been triaged, the process of reevaluating the victims begins. All of the victims should be reevaluated for changes in status. This may also be accomplished by other rescuers; however, they will be—at least initially—occupied with treating victims designated as immediate and preparing them for transport. Those victims designated as immediate may deteriorate and become expectant. If so, only comfort measures should be given and, if possible, victims should be moved to an area designated for expectant victims. Victims designated as delayed may now be immediate or victims designated as immediate but waiting for transportation may now need to be transported ahead of others also designated as immediate.[3,4]

Many of the victims presenting for treatment in the field or the hospital will be very anxious. Many of them will not be injured or in the case of a hazardous material incident, not be contaminated. Their presence will complicate triage and add significantly to the number of victims. These victims will still need to be triaged and treated. Their anxiety may disguise underlying concerns needing more significant care.[3]

Although a few triage systems have been developed, the ones most commonly used are the START or (simple triage, rapid treatment) system for adults and the Jump START system for children.[3,22]

START System

The **START** system was developed by Huag Hospital and the Newport Beach Fire Department. It is designed to allow personnel with limited medical knowledge and skill to triage victims in 60 seconds or less per victim. The system evaluates victims based on four criteria: can he respond and walk, how fast are his respirations, what is his perfusion status, and what is his mental status **(see Fig. 2–4, Table 2–4)**.

- **First:** All **walking wounded,** those who can get up and walk to a designated area, are classified as minor. These victims should be reevaluated often. Those who are not able to move to this area should be evaluated by the person or persons performing triage.

Combined START/JumpSTART Triage Algorithm

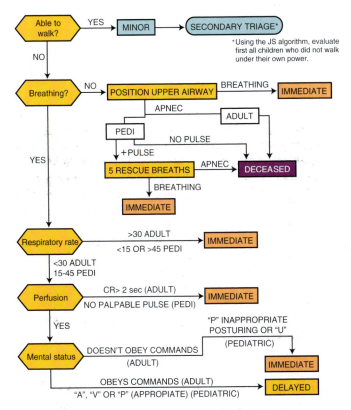

FIGURE 2–4. This algorithm depicts the START and Jump START triage systems.

- **Second:** Evaluate the victim's breathing. If the victim is not breathing, reposition the airway. If they do not begin to breathe on their own, they are classified as deceased, no other assessment is made.
- **Third:** Evaluate how quickly the victim is breathing. Respiratory rates over 30/min are classified as immediate and the rescuer moves on to the next victim. Respiratory rates under 30/min should then be evaluated for perfusion.

TABLE 2–4   START Triage Method for Adults

ASSESS	TRIAGE
1. CAN VICTIM RESPOND AND WALK?	
All who can walk around	Are classified as minor. Reevaluate often. Move on.
If victim cannot walk	Continue to assessment 2.
2. HOW FAST ARE RESPIRATIONS?	
If victim is not breathing	Reposition airway. If still not breathing classify as deceased, end assessment, move on.
If victim begins to breathe check respiration rate (RR)	
RR more than 30/min	Classify as immediate and move on.
RR less than 30/min	Continue to assessment 3.
3. WHAT IS THE PERFUSION STATUS?	
Check radial pulse and capillary refill	
If capillary refill longer than 2 seconds or no radial pulse	Tag victim as immediate; control obvious bleeding; move on.
If radial pulse in present and capillary refill is shorter than 2 seconds	Continue to assessment 4.
4. WHAT IS THE MENTAL STATUS?	
Ask victim to follow simple command (e.g., squeeze my finger, tell me your name)	
Victims who cannot follow simple commands	Tag as immediate.
Victims who can follow simple commands	Tag as delayed.

- **Fourth:** Evaluate for perfusion. The rescuer should check the victim's radial pulse or capillary refill. If the victim's capillary refill is longer than 2 seconds or there is no radial pulse, then tag the victim as immediate, quickly attempt to control obvious bleeding, and move on to the next victim.

- **Fifth:** Evaluate the mental status of the victim. When the radial pulse is present or the capillary refill is shorter than 2 seconds, evaluate the victim's mental status by asking the victim to follow a few simple commands such as squeeze my fingers and then let go or tell me your name and where you are. Victims who cannot follow simple commands are tagged as immediate. Those who meet all of the criteria are tagged as delayed.[3,23]

Jump START System

The **Jump START** system was developed by Lou E. Romig, MD, FAAP, FACEP of Team Life Support Inc. It uses criteria similar to those in the START system with adaptations for children **(see Fig. 2–4, Table 2–5).**

- **First:** As with the START system, all **walking wounded** are tagged as minor. Secondary triage or a focused reevaluation should be performed often on these victims.
  - When performing secondary triage and reevaluation, infants should be evaluated first. Each remaining victim should be evaluated according to breathing, respiratory rate, pulse, and AVPU (alert, verbal, or responsive only to pain, posturing or unresponsive).

- **Second:** If the victim is not breathing, reposition the airway. If they begin to breathe, tag them as immediate and move on, if they do not, then assess the victim's pulse. If there is no pulse, the victim is deceased.
  - If there is a pulse, but the victim is not breathing, perform five rescue breaths. If the victim remains apneic, they are tagged as deceased; if they begin to breathe they are tagged as immediate.

- **Third:** Those victims who are breathing should be evaluated for the rate of respirations. Those victims with rates

TABLE 2–5   The JUMPStart Triage Method for Use With Children

ASSESS	TRIAGE
1. CAN VICTIM RESPOND AND WALK?	
All who can walk around	Are classified as minor; secondary evaluation often. Move on.
If victim cannot walk	Continue to assessment 2.
2. IS VICTIM BREATHING?	
If victim is not breathing	Reposition airway. If breathing begins classify as immediate, and move on. If still not breathing check pulse. If no pulse classify as deceased. If there is a pulse but no breathing perform 5 rescue breathes. If no breathing classify as deceased, move on.
If victim begins to breathe check respiration rate (RR)	If breathing begins classify as immediate and check rate.
RR more than 36/min	Classify as immediate and move on.
RR less than 15/min	Classify and immediate and move on.
RR between 15 and 36/min	Continue to assessment 3.
3. WHAT IS THE PERFUSION STATUS?	
Check pulse	
If no palpable pulse	Classify as immediate.
With palpable pulse	Continue to assessment 4.
4. WHAT IS THE MENTAL STATUS?	
If victim alert and responds to verbal stimuli appropriately	Classify as delayed.
If they only respond to pain, are posturing, or if unresponsive	Tag as immediate.

below 15 or above 36 should be tagged as immediate and move on. Those with rates between 15 and 36 should be evaluated for perfusion.

- **Fourth:** Evaluate the victim's pulse. If they do not have a palpable pulse they are classified as immediate.
- **Fifth:** Those with a palpable pulse should be evaluated for mental status. If the victim is alert and responds to verbal stimuli appropriately, they are tagged as delayed. If they inappropriately respond only to pain, are posturing, or if they are unresponsive, they are tagged as immediate.[24]

These processes must be performed quickly. Children and adults are not separated and should be triaged in the order that they are found. Start with the person nearest you and move to the next when you finish. The triage systems are designed to take less than 1 minute per person. Even at 1 minute, if there is only one person performing triage and there are 60 victims, triage alone will take more than 1 hour. If there are multiple personnel performing triage, there needs to be one person who is directing the operation.

Overtriage and Undertriage

It is important to touch on the concepts of over and under-triage. Undertriage occurs when victims are classified as minor when they should be delayed or classified as delayed when they should be immediate. Acceptable rates for undertriage are near 5%. This is kept low because if victims are undertriaged, they are not receiving the life-saving care required by their level of acuity. Victims tagged delayed when they should be tagged immediate may die needlessly. In the chaotic world of a disaster, this may happen. Overtriage occurs when a victim is classified as immediate when they should be classified as delayed. Although more acceptable than undertriage, this utilizes resources that should be used for more serious victims. Acceptable rates for overtriage are much higher in an effort to avoid undertriage. Rates of 50% have been acceptable. In addition, as a result of the possibility for rapid decompensation, overtriage is far more acceptable than undertriage especially with children.[3]

Summary

Triage is a daily part of life in the pre-hospital and hospital setting. During MCIs or disaster events, the systems change. In the day-to-day setting, the most critical victims or patients requiring large amounts of resources, even if there is a doubtful positive outcome, are seen and treated first whereas during an MCI or disaster they are kept comfortable while treatment is provided for those with a greater chance of survival. Triage is the difficult task of sorting victims so that the maximum number of victims are treated and will survive with the limited resources available. Although hospital and field triage differ during an MCI or disaster in some aspects, both have the essential task of moving victims who are most in need and have the best chance of survival to the most appropriate location or facility for the most appropriate treatment. It must be done quickly and decisively; treatment in the field is provided by those rescuers and providers who give care after triage has been completed. Who they treat or transport first is dictated by the person performing triage. Victims waiting for transportation or treatment should be retriaged often for changes in their condition. Each victim must be tagged for both identification and documentation of treatment.

Well-organized triage, even done quickly, may consume a significant amount of manpower and time, depending on the size of the event. It is, however, necessary to ensure the best positive outcomes for the most victims.

REFERENCES

1. Larkin GL, Arnold J. Ethical considerations in emergency planning, preparedness, and response to acts of terrorism. *Journal of Prehospital and Disaster Medicine.* 2003;18(3):170–178.

2. Severance, HW. Mass-casualty victim "surge" management. Preparing for bombings and blast-related injuries with possibility of hazardous materials exposure. *North Carolina Medical Journal.* 2002;63(5):242–246.

3. Hogan DE, Jonathan L, eds. *Disaster Medicine.* Philadelphia, PA: Lippincott Williams & Wilkins; 2002, 432.

4. Kennedy K, Aghababian RV, Gans L, Lewis CP. Triage: techniques and applications in decision making. *Annals of Emergency Medicine*. 1996;28(2):136–144.

5. Roccaforte JD, Cushman JG. Disaster preparedness, triage, and surge capacity for hospital definitive care areas: optimizing outcomes when demands exceed resources. *Anesthesiology Clinics*. 2007;25(1):161–177.

6. Born CT, Briggs SM, Ciraulo DL, et al. Disasters and mass casualties: I. General principles of response and management. [see comment]. *Journal of the American Academy of Orthopaedic Surgeons*. 2007;15(7):388–396.

7. Cotter S. Treatment area considerations for mass casualty incidents. *Emergency Medical Services*. 2006;35(2):48–51.

8. Irvin CB, Atas, JG. Management of evacuee surge from a disaster area: solutions to avoid non-emergent, emergency department visits. *Journal of Prehospital and Disaster Medicine*. 2007;22(3):220–223.

9. Grimaldi ME. Ethical decisions in times of disaster: choices healthcare workers must make. *Journal of Trauma Nursing*. 2007;14(3):163–164.

10. Hotchkin DL, Rubinson L. Modified critical care and treatment space considerations for mass casualty critical illness and injury. *Respiratory Care*. 2008;53(1):67–74; discussion 74–77.

11. Sztajnkrycer MD, Madsen BE, Alejandro Baez A. Unstable ethical plateaus and disaster triage. *Emergency Medicine Clinics of North America*. 2006;24(3):749–768.

12. Brousseau DC, Mistry RD, Alessandrini EA. Methods of categorizing emergency department visit urgency: a survey of pediatric emergency medicine physicians. *Pediatric Emergency Care*. 2006; 22(9): 635–639.

13. Lynch EL, Thomas TL. Pediatric considerations in chemical exposures: are we prepared? *Pediatric Emergency Care*. 2004; 20(3):198–208.

14. Garner A. Documentation and tagging of casualties in multiple casualty incidents. *Emergency Medicine*. 2003;15(5–6): 475–479.

15. Hoey BA, Schwab CW. Level I center triage and mass casualties. *Clinical Orthopaedics and Related Research*. 2004;(422): 23–29.

16. Fry EA, Lenert LA. MASCAL: RFID tracking of patients, staff and equipment to enhance hospital response to mass casualty events. AMIA Annual Symposium Proceedings 2005; 261–265.

17. Farmer JC, Carlton PK Jr. Providing critical care during a disaster: the interface between disaster response agencies and hospitals. *Critical Care Medicine*. 2006;34(3 Suppl): S56–S59.

18. Hale JF. Managing a disaster scene and multiple casualties before help arrives. *Critical Care Nursing Clinics of North America*. 2008;20(1): 91–102.

19. Farmer JC, Carlton PK Jr. Hospital disaster medical response: aligning everyday requirements with emergency casualty care. *World Hospitals and Health Services*. 2005;41(2):21–24.

20. Furbee PM, Coben JH, Smyth SK, et al. Realities of rural emergency medical services disaster preparedness. *Journal of Prehospital and Disaster Medicine*. 2006;21(2 Suppl):64–70.

21. Zoraster RM, Chidester C, Koenig W. Field triage and patient maldistribution in a mass-casualty incident. *Journal of Prehospital and Disaster Medicine*. 2007;22(3):224–229.

22. Gebhart ME, Pence R. START triage: does it work? *Journal of Disaster Management and Response*. 2007;5(3):68–73.

23. Department of Defense. NUCLEAR WEAPONS EFFECTS TECHNOLOGY, Military Critical Technologies List (MCTL). Editor. 2008.

24. Romig L. JumpSTART Triage. 2008. Available at: http://www. jumpstarttriage.com/. Accessed June 23, 2008.

Preparedness for the Hospital and Other Institutions

Introduction

This chapter will discuss the preparations that hospitals and other similar institutions will need to examine and implement to prepare for and respond to disasters. This is a broad topic that cannot be completely covered in this book, but key topics will be presented that will enable health-care institutions to begin to establish a comprehensive and realistic preparedness plan. The first section deals with mitigation and preparation. It is subdivided into sections covering the stockpiling of supplies, licensure concerns, and communication issues. The chapter goes on to discuss surge issues and the response of the hospital or institution to a disaster. It is important to note that disasters may be local, relatively small, mass casualty incidents (MCIs), or they may be extensive, regional incidents with far-reaching affects and extensive response locally, as well as a state and federal response. The institution's disaster plan should be able to respond to both **(see Fig. 3–1).**

Hospital disaster planning should be done through a committee process with all aspects of the hospital participating. Nursing is a large part of any hospital or clinic and nurse practitioners (NP) and other advance practice nurses (APNs) are playing an increasingly important role in these settings. It is very important that both be a part of hospital disaster planning and response. Nursing administration should support this by providing time for nurses and NPs to be present at these meetings and encouraging training to improve both planning and response. Administration should also support adequate supplies and equipment to facilitate this response in as safe a manner as possible given the austere circumstances of a disaster.

Nursing education must prepare undergraduate students with an understanding of disaster preparation and planning and continuing education should build upon that base. This training should be extensive and provide a deep understanding of the realities and restrictions of preparation. Students and practicing nurses, NPs and APNs should be aware of the nature of disaster response, changes in standards of care, and the realities of the austere climate within disaster response. Without this awareness, conflicts, misunderstandings, and unmet expectations will severely limit the effectiveness of the response.

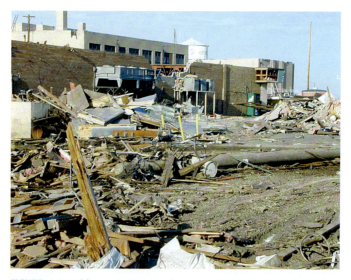

FIGURE 3–1. Hoisington, Kansas, April 26, 2001. The Hoisington tornado damaged the high school, a small shopping center, the hospital, and hundreds of homes in a matter of minutes. Hospitals are susceptible to storms, earthquake, and other manmade and natural disasters. A well thought out plan is essential, but even these may fail. *Photo By Dave Saville/FEMA News Photo.*

Institutional preparedness is complex on many levels. In general, institutions should be prepared to be self sufficient for at least 72 to 96 hours without outside intervention and aid. (This requirement varies by accrediting, credentialing, and advising bodies.) Although there may be private and government sources of aid available, there may be concerns with infrastructure, transportation, and other practical issues affecting its distribution and delivery. Local sources of food, water, linens, and other supplies will be affected by the same physical concerns affecting a hospital or clinic. Bridges and roads that feed an area may be clogged from damage or debris. The aid available may not reach the institutions that need it.[1–3]

Before the Hurricane Katrina disaster, one hospital in New Orleans had prepared by developing a disaster plan that included protocols, triggers for implementation, and stockpiles of food, water, and supplies near the hospital. As the hurricane approached, the plan was put into effect. Personnel were to be prepared to stay at the hospital until they were released after the disaster. A second team, known as the recovery team, was to take their place when it was safe and they were able to report to the hospital. Supplies were moved to the hospital from a nearby storage facility, and as the hurricane struck, the full hospital disaster plan was put into effect.

WHY IS IT IMPORTANT To Have Hospital Preparedness?

Like personal preparedness plans, hospitals should be prepared to survive on their own for 3 to 4 days. There may be sources of outside aid, but these may be delayed by the needs of other institutions, damage or impassable infrastructure, or simply the scope of the disaster itself. Without adequate food, water, pharmaceuticals, and other supplies, patients and staff will suffer and outcomes will be less positive. Being prepared to meet the needs of staff, patients, and the influx of victims from the disaster is also the ethical responsibility of the hospital to the community as an extension of the daily care provided by the institution.

As the storm passed, flooding from the nearby broken levies caused the hospital auxiliary generator to fail and severely limited outside access to the hospital. The result was limited electrical power and an inability to evacuate patients or resupply the hospital. A few portable generators provided some electrical power. Air conditioning was not functioning and temperatures rapidly rose to more than 100 degrees. Food for the patients was adequate, however because of cafeteria flooding, staff meals consisted of a half cup of cold canned food. Only bottled water was available. Hand sanitizer was the most popular form of personal hygiene; some staff used it for bathing. Toothpaste was not available. Portable toilets soon overflowed; the regular toilets were not functional. Some floors used buckets and placed waste in plastic bags for disposal, on other floors, it simply piled up or stairwells were used. Evacuating patients from floor to floor required up to six staff members, moving boarded patients, down stairwells in the dark. The families of the on-duty staff came to the hospital for safety during the storm, which added to the stress placed on the system. Pets were not to be included; however, some staff brought their pets anyway. Eventually, all patients and staff were evacuated using boats and large tractor trailer trucks as ambulances.

Although this hospital had what may be considered a realistic and well thought out disaster plan, circumstances changed and unforeseen problems negated some of the preparations. They had planned for meeting the needs of the hospital, staff, and patients but within 24 hours flooding caused a power outage, made food preparation nearly impossible, and incapacitated the sewer system. Air conditioning failed, sewage backed up, and food needed to be rationed. When evacuation was possible, it was carried out through dark stairwells into unconventional vehicles.

Disaster plans for hospitals and other health-care sites must be realistic and updated regularly. They must consider the risks the institution may face and they must be flexible enough to adapt to problems as they occur. Each institution also should realize that it cannot be prepared for every possibility. In the previous example, adequate preparations were made for personnel, food, water, other supplies, and power; extensive and sustained flooding negated many aspects of these preparations. Institutions will need to adapt as much as possible and should, in future preparations, consider changing the plan to meet the additional challenges. Health-care providers and institutions have a responsibility to prepare to meet the needs of the hospital, the staff, and patients during a disaster; however, it is not possible to be prepared for all eventualities.

Disaster Planning

The requirements and considerations for preparing for 96 hours without outside aid include:

- **Developing a hospital or institutional command structure.** The community will be using some form of the incident command system (ICS). An emergency operations center will be established with an incident commander exerting control over the area. Other sections will be established under his or her control including: planning, operations, logistics, and finance with small functional teams working in each area. Similarly, the institution must establish a command structure with one commander overseeing section leaders or commanders for each area. Although it may not be realistic to keep teams to the three to seven members established in the ICS, teams should be kept as small and functional as possible with defined tasks to avoid confusion.[4]

- **Having food, water, medications, linens, supplies, and other needs for all patients and staff for a hospital that may be serving many more injured and ill than there would be under normal circumstances.** Purchasing, storing, and maintaining such a cache for even a small institution is a daunting endeavor **(see Fig. 3–2)**. Financial resources for the initial outlay and continued renewal of this cache is significant for institutions that, at best, operate with a less than 5% margin. It also requires a large, safe storage facility; space that most likely is needed for other worthy projects.

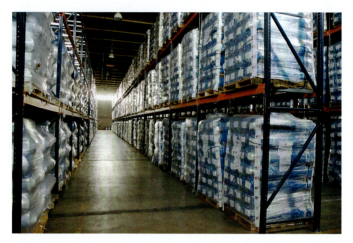

FIGURE 3–2. Lufkin, Texas, September 2, 2008. Pallets of water sit in a warehouse in Lufkin, Texas. *Photo by Patsy Lynch/FEMA.*

- **Having water and power for patient and staff needs such as cleaning linens, food preparation, and other needs.** Public utilities may not be functioning. A generator will provide some power but may not be able to meet all power needs throughout the institution. The location of the generator may place it at risk of damage from flooding or other disaster-related occurrences. The need for fuel and service also will add to the financial commitment and storage needs.[1,2,5–7]

WHY IS IT IMPORTANT **To Realize Hospital Preparedness Is Difficult?**

Hospital preparedness is a balance of financial concerns and the responsibility of the institution to meet the needs of disaster victims, the community, and the staff of the institution. With hospitals operating with only small margins (little capital and income compared with operating costs and other expenses), there is little or no extra money available to spend on something that may never happen.

- **Having a plan for functioning while short staffed with above normal numbers of sick and injured patients presenting for treatment.**
- **Developing protocols and triggers for implementation for alternative standards of care.** Nurses may need to act in the role of physicians, practitioners and physicians will act beyond their specialties and roles. Areas of the hospital will need to be protected so they are available for those who need them most. For instance, radiology and surgery will be used only for those who absolutely need the intervention most. Security personnel will need to direct the flow of patients, victims, families, media, staff, volunteers, and others to different locations and control their movement throughout their stay. They will also need to provide physical security for staff and patients in a chaotic world with less than normal staffing levels.[1,2]
- **Having a plan for volunteers and organizations who will respond to help treat patients.** Nurses, practitioners, physicians, and other licensed personnel both from nearby and from other states will offer help. Their help may be desperately needed, but without verification procedures in place, can the hospital use them to the fullest? Some states now have agreements in place to honor other state's licensure and there is a move to extend this nationally, but this may remain an issue for some time to come. Nonlicensed personnel also will offer help. Where and how will they be used? Outside organizations may have large tents or other equipment. The hospital needs to make itself aware of community resources that may assist in its response.
- **Establish an effective intrahospital or institution communication system and back-up alternatives.** Communication between the units of the hospital, the floors, and the command structure is essential for the hospital to function. Depending on the size and impact of the disaster, phones and other established modes of communication may not be functional. Other means of communication may include radios or a simple system of runners.

> **WHY IS IT IMPORTANT** **To Have Protocols?**
>
> Protocols for credentialing volunteer staff and for treating victims and patients during austere times are vitally important to protect medical and nursing staff and those being treated. Protocols allow quick, yet efficient credentialing of professional volunteers from the local area and the outside who offer aid during a disaster. In the treatment arena, it allows nursing staff to function to their fullest potential under guidelines set in advance. They also provide some liability protection.

- **Having protocols to ensure communication and response procedures.** Law enforcement, fire service, emergency medical services, and other professional organizations will be both stretched and desperately needed at the hospital. Are lines of communication set up between the community's disaster response and the various health-care institutions in the area? Discussions need to take place before a disaster strikes to decide which patients go to which institutions and how many victims each institution can handle. Communication systems need to be compatible so that community agencies are able to speak directly to the hospital even if the phone lines are disabled.[2,8]

In the end, institutions must have realistic, comprehensive, disaster plans and it must be practiced and tested. Difficult questions must be asked and answered. It is not possible to prepare for all eventualities, but for those that institutions know may occur, they should have some preparations.

Mitigation

Mitigation is key to institutional preparedness. Stockpiling supplies and establishing protocols will allow the institution to respond to disasters and mass casualty events in a more organized and effective manner. It involves establishing organizational structures such as lines of authority and developing relationships and their supporting structures with the community and others. Institutional mitigation involves a significant investment of time, money, and commitment from everyone in the institution, especially top management, if it is to succeed.[1,2]

Stockpiling

Food, water, supplies, equipment, everything necessary for a hospital, clinic, or other health-care institution to function on a day-to-day basis is necessary for it to function during a disaster. With a large influx of victims, more food, water, and other necessities will be needed than under normal circumstances.[5] Although state and federal government support exist to help provide for these necessities, in a disaster they will be in short supply and delivery delays may occur. If an institution does not have enough water, food, medications, and other needs to provide for patients and victims who are already in distress, increases in morbidity and mortality will result.

Stockpiling supplies requires a large protected storage area with easy access from the facility. Such warehousing is difficult. It needs to be a substantial structure that will withstand severe weather such as high winds or heavy snows. Temperature should be controlled to protect sensitive medications and other supplies from freezing or extreme heat. It should be well above flood plains and other hazards such as industrial hazards that may become a factor in the event of a disaster **(see Fig. 3-3).** It should be close to or within easy access to the institution without the potential loss of sensitive infrastructure such as bridges. Stockpiling requires well trained personnel to manage the operation. Large quantities of various supplies are of no use if they are not organized and accessible quickly. Warehousing on this level is expensive and difficult.[5,7]

Purchasing Agreements

Purchasing agreements may provide an alternative to large stockpiling needs, but they do have limitations. Purchasing agreements are contracts between an institution and its suppliers that state that the supplier will deliver to the institution needed supplies at either a preset price or the current market value in the event of a disaster. Suppliers provide supplies to various institutions; they have access to large warehoused

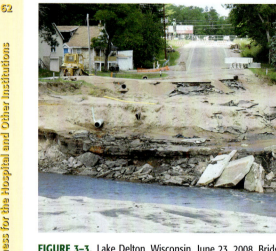

FIGURE 3–3. Lake Delton, Wisconsin, June 23, 2008. Bridges, roads, and houses are damaged at Lake Delton as flood waters compromised a dam that eroded the lake basin and walls, draining the lake into the nearby Wisconsin River. Damage to local infrastructure may compromise the hospital's ability to access warehouses and other outside sources of aid in a disaster. *Photo by Robert Kaufmann/FEMA.*

supplies; and are better equipped to warehouse large quantities of food, water, medications, and other needs. There are limitations to these arrangements. If the supplier does not have the supplies for delivery, they cannot deliver them. It is also likely that purchasing agreements will be made with other institutions in the area. This places the responsibility on the supplier for warehousing and making available large quantities of supplies for many of the institutions in the area. Transportation of the needed supplies is another concern. Any warehouse located near the institution will likely be affected by the same disaster. Infrastructure may be clogged with debris or blocked by damage making deliveries difficult or impossible.[5,7]

Pharmaceuticals

When establishing stockpiles of supplies, pharmaceuticals require special consideration **(see Fig. 3–4).** It is important to note that the need for the standard formulary will not diminish

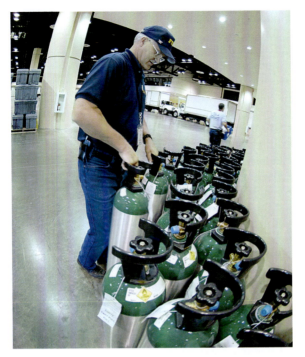

FIGURE 3–4. A warehouse worker tracks oxygen and other supplies with a bar code scanner. Organization of supplies and pharmaceuticals requires a significant amount of space and manpower but is essential to preparedness. *Photo by Jocelyn Augustino/FEMA.*

during or after a disaster. Chronic illnesses will not go away because of the disaster; high blood pressure, diabetes, and other diseases will still need to be treated.[9] Beyond these medications, a risk analysis should identify medications that need to be stockpiled.[10–12]

A list of considerations would include:

- Weather related
  - Trauma from high winds and collapsed structures
    - Antibiotics
    - Tetanus prophylaxis
    - Local and general anesthetics
    - Pain medications

- Flooding
  - Antibiotics
  - Tetanus prophylaxis
  - Local anesthetics
- Terrorism
  - Biological
    - Antibiotics and antivirals
    - Antitoxins
    - Fluids and electrolytes
  - Chemical
    - Beta-agonist inhalers
    - Fluids and electrolytes
    - Cyanide treatment
    - Burn treatments
    - Sedatives
    - Pain medications
  - Oximes, atropine, or pralidoxime choride, Pyridostigmine bromide, and benzodiazepines for nerve agents[13]
  - Radiation
    - Burn treatments
    - Prussian blue, ammonium phosphate
    - Ca gluconate
    - Na or Ca bicarbonate
    - Fluids and electrolytes
    - Pain medications

The amount of each medication each institution should have on hand is difficult to answer. Some medications, for instance those associated with radiation injuries, may never be used by many institutions. Other medications would not be used in the amounts needed for a bioterrorism attack, such as respiratory botulism. Botulism does occur and an event may involve several individuals; however, it is unlikely that the number of victims institutions are prepared to treat would equal the number who would choose to present in the event of a terrorist aerosolized botulism attack. Stockpiling large amounts of some medications that would never be used may not be prudent.

There are outside sources of pharmaceuticals and some supplies. The Strategic National Stockpile (SNS) is operated through the Centers for Disease Control and Prevention under the Department of Health and Human Services and is designed to provide medications, chemical antidotes, antitoxins, medical supplies, and airway supplies.[11] Push packages are designed and stored in a way that allows them to be loaded immediately onto trucks or aircraft and delivered anywhere in the United States within 12 hours. They are followed by vendor managed inventories (VMI) with more specific medications after the need is known. These would arrive in 24 to 48 hours. If the agent or agents are known, the VMI should be requested first. These supplies must be requested by the state's governor's office. The supplies are delivered to the state for further distribution to local communities. The technical advisory response unit (TARU) responds with the "12 hour push package" and remains to assist with distribution of the supplies. These medications and supplies are provided at no charge to the state **(see Fig. 3-5)**.[12,14,15]

This source of medications and supplies depend on transportation to first reach the state and then the local communities where the incident is occurring. This transportation

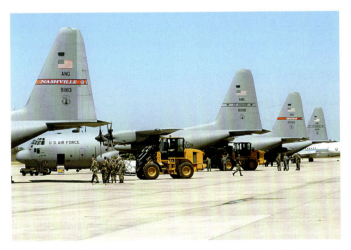

FIGURE 3–5. Gulfport, Mississippi, September 7, 2005. Cargo aircraft from all over the United States bring supplies including medical supplies into the National Guard airfield in Gulfport, Mississippi. Hurricane Katrina caused shortages of supplies throughout the gulf coast of Mississippi. *Photo by Mark Wolfe/FEMA.*

WHY IS IT IMPORTANT **To Keep a Strategic National Stockpile?**

The Strategic National Stockpile (SNS) makes available Push Packages of medications and supplies including airway supplies for delivery to any state within 12 to 24 hours in the event of a disaster. This is followed by Vendor Managed Inventories (VMI) designed to meet the specific needs of the incident. A Technical Advisory Response Unit (TARU) accompanies the VMI to assist in distribution from the state to the local communities. The packages are delivered to the state capital and then distributed to the areas of need. This distribution may be limited by damaged or clogged infrastructure but should allow supplies to reach areas of need within 48 to 72 hours.

depends on a functioning transportation system with intact infrastructure. Roads and bridges, airports, and other aspects of the broad transportation system may be affected by the incident either directly by being damaged or indirectly by people fleeing the area. In the event of a terrorist attack, transportation infrastructure may be targeted specifically to limit and delay the response to a biological, chemical, or nuclear event. Because of this, institutions should not see the SNS as the sole source of their response. An adequate amount of medications must be on hand to attempt to treat illnesses and injuries or in the event of a biological terrorist attack or pandemic, attempt to contain initial outbreak.[10–12,15,16]

Supplies and Equipment

As with pharmaceuticals, the risk assessment performed by the institution will identify disaster-related needs. There may be some instances in which the hospital is able to discharge some of its patients to make room for disaster victims; however, most patients will not be able to be discharged. Elective procedures may be cancelled, but it is likely that more procedures will be performed related to the disaster. Linens, dressings, IV tubing, syringes, medicine cups, drinking cups, plates, utensils, office supplies, in short everything used on a daily basis will show a significant increase in use.[5]

Each type of event will require specific items. For instance:

- Severe viral pandemics will likely require ventilators, airway supplies, and isolation equipment.
- Tornados, severe storms, and earthquakes will likely require trauma and surgical supplies.
- Extreme cold would require patient warming equipment, blankets, and warming units for intravenous fluids.
- Terrorist attacks would require several differing types of equipment from trauma and surgical supplies to decontamination equipment and ventilators.

At least some of the events the institution will face will limit or stop access to necessary public utilities. Auxiliary generators will provide some power but will require fuel storage. Although it may be possible to replenish this fuel, conditions may make it impossible to receive additional fuel for days. Water may be cut off completely or simply be contaminated. Depending on the contamination, it may be possible to use it to clean and wash linens but not be potable; there would need to be another source of drinking water. Natural gas may be cut off requiring alternative methods of cooking or providing heat during cold weather. The lack of air conditioning and ventilation will be a concern. Sanitation may be a concern. If the sanitary sewers are not functional, portable or chemical toilets will be necessary. These toilets will fill

WHY IS IT IMPORTANT To Have Utility Planning?

The Joint Commission has stated that part of an institution's disaster plan must include steps to ensure that utility needs are met in the event of a loss of public utilities. Water, gas, and electricity are essential for normal operations within the hospital. During extremes in weather, hospitals will become unbearably hot or cold in a short time without heating and air-conditioning. Many patient needs, such as ventilators, require electricity to operate for extended periods. Planning to include sources of water, gas for cooking and other needs, and electrical power need to be realistic and comprehensive. Problems such as auxiliary generators located in areas that may flood or be susceptible to other damage must be considered.

quickly so alternatives may be necessary such as something as simple as a bucket with a plastic bag or a bedside commode with a plastic bag liner. If it is a large institution with hundreds of staff and victims, this solution will fail quickly.

Spare supplies must be stored near the institution in a building secure enough to survive whatever concerns the institution may be at risk for. If there is enough warning before the event, the supplies should be moved into the facility. If not, the storage area must be able to be accessed safely during the event. Equipment needed to transport the supplies also will need to be available and able to function in spite of the event.

Licensure and Staffing Issues

Health-care providers are licensed within the state where they work. Nurses, nurse practitioners, physician assistants, and physicians are further credentialed within each institution. The process within the institution may involve drug screening, background checks for felonies, additional checks for child abuse, finger printing, physicals, and educational and reference checks. In addition, there are liability concerns.[17] Although these credentialing and licensure issues make it very difficult for volunteers to help during a disaster; they are necessary.

It is unreasonable to use the traditional credentialing methods during a disaster. Communication systems may not be functional and there is not enough time to check the licensure, education, and experience of those who offer help. Waves of victims will be presenting to the hospital for care. Many of the hospital's regular workforce may be unable to report to work thus creating more staffing issues. Any volunteers who offer help will be difficult to turn away, It may be possible to verify some information when the volunteer presents, for instance, the licensure of physicians, nurse practitioners, physician assistants can be verified by contacting the state licensure boards; this requires an Internet connection or phone line. Holding the paper copy of a license does not verify that the license has not been revoked. Steps may be taken to credential volunteers before a disaster but this can only occur if the potential volunteers are known.[18]

Plans should be developed by the credentialing staff of the institution to provide emergency credentials for nursing and medical staff. They will need to consider beforehand what credentialing information will be required from volunteers, and what services they will be permitted to perform. If only paper licenses are available, the volunteer may be allowed to perform only limited services. If there is time to verify more, more may be permitted. If possible, lists of potential volunteers may be established during the planning stage. These potential volunteers may be made up of nurses and physicians or other personnel who have left or retired from the hospital. Others may include personnel from other hospitals or institutions, nurses and general practitioners from private practices.[19] There are problems that may make this plan less functional.[20–22] Retired personnel may not have the stamina to work the long intense hours required. They and other volunteers will not be familiar with operations and protocols of the hospital. They will be unfamiliar with authority structures and, depending on how long they have been retired, their skills dull. Other volunteers from private practices or other hospitals will be busy with victims presenting to their facilities and may not be available to supplement staffing. Volunteers may come from outside the area, but there may be no reasonable way to anticipate who they would be and verify licensure or credentials prior to the event.[18] Some states have developed multistate compacts that would allow some health-care providers to work in other states within the compact. There also is a move by the National State Boards of Nursing to allow licenses to be accepted across the country.

Staffing needs will more likely be met if the family needs of the hospital's staff are met. Providing shelter for staff families and pets will decrease the potential of staff reporting off because of the need to care for their families. Many institutions' disaster planning includes provisions for staff's families allowing staff to report with their families and pets. Preplanning will help to provide space, food, water, and staff to care for those family members and pets who require personal care. This is particularly important for the very

WHY IS IT IMPORTANT To Provide for the Needs of Staff?

Medical, nursing, and other professional and nonprofessional staff will be affected by the same disaster that affects the hospital. They must be trained to prepare for their own needs and those of the families to avoid being so overcome by the disaster that they cannot perform their duties within the health-care system. The hospital should also look to provide for the needs of their staff by providing refuge and care for families and pets. This places an additional burden on the institution but allows the staff to care for others knowing that the needs of their families are being met. The staffing needs of the hospital will most likely be met during a disaster if the staff is well trained in disaster response and the needs of family and pets are provided for by the institution.

young, the elderly, and any pets. Providing staff to care for and meet these needs will add to the burdens experienced by the institution during a disaster, but will allow staff to commit to the institution.[23,24]

There are federal sources of staffing. The Disaster Medical Assistance Teams (DMAT), pharmacy emergency response team (PERT), and the United States Public Health Service Commissioned Corps may be deployed to provide extra staffing[25,26] **(see Figs. 3–6 and 3–7).** DMAT is able to provide self-standing hospitals or personnel to staff clinics and shelters. The U.S. Public Health Service also can be deployed to help staff hospitals and clinics in stricken areas. These resources are limited.

In addition to professional staff needs, the institution may need volunteers to help with patient transport, food services, janitorial, and other needs. Nonprofessional volunteers may be able to help in these areas. It is important to note that if these volunteers are untrained, that is unfamiliar with the hospital and its realities in a disaster situation, they may become overwhelmed or may be limited in their ability to respond.[18] It should also be noted that they may not have gone through the normal background screening normally performed on anybody who works in the hospital.

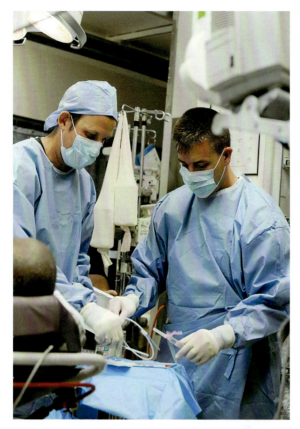

FIGURE 3–6. Galveston Island, Texas, September 19, 2008. Members of the Disaster Medical Assistance Team (DMAT) attempt to put a central line in a patient who has come to the hospital for care. DMAT personnel can provide needed services in a disaster, greatly increasing the surge capacity of the local medical community. *Photo by Jocelyn Augustino/FEMA.*

Institutions can ask for volunteers before the event. As with the professional staffing list mentioned earlier, the hospital can ask for potential volunteers from the local and surrounding community and create a list. People on this list could then attend regular training sessions and be involved in annual drills. Background checks also can be performed. This has the benefit of creating a trained volunteer workforce familiar with disaster

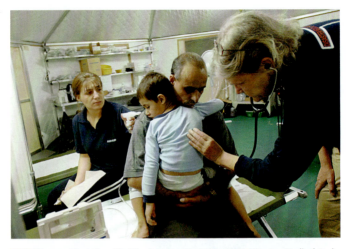

FIGURE 3–7. Plantation, Florida, October 28, 2005. FEMA Disaster Medical Assistance Team (DMAT) member Dr. Allene Jackson from Oklahoma One, listens to the breathing of Karim Alabboad who is being held by his father Saoud Alabboad while his mother Samira Shalan helps with a breathing treatment for asthma. The DMAT is set up next to Westside Regional Hospital to help with the increase of patients to the emergency room due to Hurricane Wilma. *Photo by Jocelyn Augustino/FEMA.*

response, hospital policy, and staff. A large list from the broad surrounding area increases the chance that some would be available during a disaster. Institutions may also integrate Community Emergency Response Teams (CERT) or other volunteer organizations from their area. CERT teams are citizens who have received light disaster response training and are organized into local volunteer response teams. Other volunteer teams may be active in the area and be capable of providing assistance. Volunteer search and rescue teams and others may be available to assist with transportation of personnel to and from the hospital, delivering medications, or other tasks within the institution. The institution should make itself aware of these local groups and their capabilities **(see Table 3–1).**

Communications

Communication concerns, both internal and external, are difficult issues with limited answers. **Internal communication**

TABLE 3–1 List of Volunteer Groups That May Provide Aid to the Hospital

LEVEL	GROUP	CONCERNS
Local	**Retired Professionals:** Retired physicians, practitioners, physician assistants, nurses, and pharmacists.	Licensure and credentials will need to be confirmed. Individuals who may not have worked for a significant period of time may have limited skills.
	Retired Nonprofessionals: People from the community who have not worked in health care.	Will have limited skills and may not be trained in disaster response so they may not be personally equipped to face the austere conditions.
	Community Emergency Response Teams (CERT): Citizen teams with light disaster training.	May or may not have any health-care experience. They have disaster response training. May be being used in areas of disaster response not directly related to patient care or not related to health care at all.
	Local Volunteer Groups: Local groups such as search and rescue groups and others.	May be well organized and trained, but may not have any disaster response training. May be being used in other areas of the disaster response.
National	**FEMA DMAT and DMORT Teams:*** Teams specifically trained and equipped in disaster response.	Well-equipped and trained teams, but will need 24 to 48 hours to respond.
	U.S. Public Health Service Commissioned Corps: Part of the U.S. Uniformed Services	Well-trained individuals who help in almost any aspect of the health-care response, but will need 24 to 48 hours to respond.

*Federal Emergency Management Agency (FEMA); Disaster Medical Assistance Teams (DMAT); Disaster Mortuary Operational Response Teams (DMORT).

is defined as communication within the hospital; from floor to floor, unit to unit, incident command center to units within the authority structure of the institution. **External communication** is defined as communication with outside organizations and authorities. This would include emergency medical services, law enforcement, fire service, outside incident command posts or emergency response groups, and state or federal agencies such as the Centers for Disease Control and Prevention. The concerns involve technology and protocols.[2,27]

Internal Communication

Communication technology has become increasingly complex. Phone systems allow for several options and enhancements but now require a separate source of power to function. Radios are limited in the frequencies they can use and building materials make it difficult for radios to be effective between floors. Solutions are expensive and may have limitations and compatibility issues with other systems. In the end, during disasters, internal communication is often carried out using runners to bring messages between floors and units.

An internal communication system must first be able to function in austere circumstances. Hard-wired systems are susceptible to damage and failure if the building is damaged. If communication systems depend on an outside power source, they will fail if the utilities are lost. If they are a combined internal and external phone system and the outside phone lines are down, the internal portion also may not be functional. Radios may be an option but should be tested before making a large investment. The systems should be functional from all major areas of the hospital to all other major areas of the hospital. An alternative may be to have a designated communications center that relays information to areas that cannot communicate directly. The radios should be able to use multiple frequencies. In a disaster, not all areas of the hospital will need to hear all of the information all the time. Radios with multiple frequencies will allow for communication to be dedicated between certain areas such as the triage area and the ED, or other areas that will need to communicate often. However, having multiple frequencies will add complexity to the system. Protocols should be established early and tested to ensure they decrease confusion and not add to it.

Designate who will talk on the radios and train them. Communication over the airwaves intimidates some people. Add to that the stress of a disaster and effective communication will falter. Communication should be clear and concise. The person calling and who they want to speak to should be communicated first. For instance: "Emergency Department, this is the Triage area" and then wait for the transmission to be acknowledged. The message itself should be thought through before the person begins to speak. Ambiguous words should not be used. Messages should be short with frequent stops to allow the receiving person to break in if there is a problem. Speak slowly; often the person on the receiving end will be writing down the information as you are speaking. Establish common commands such as "prepare to copy" meaning write this down, or "stand by" meaning wait a minute, or "affirmative" or "negative" for yes and no. Use the military or local emergency services alphabet when speaking individual letter, such as "Echo Kilo Gulf" for EKG or Delta for "D" so it is not confused with "P" or "E" **(see Table 3–2).** Utilize military time references such as 0900 for 9 a.m. to remove any ambiguity. These codes are not intended to block information from people listening in; they are intended to eliminate ambiguous communication. They only work if practiced regularly.[2] The Joint Commission requires two drills each year (one of which may be a table-top exercise that may not use all of the systems and protocols); however, adding smaller more frequent drills will not add a significant cost in time or money and will ensure a more functional disaster response.

External Communication

External communication requires close coordination with the broader community.[1] An ideal system will allow for emergency communication with all aspects of the community's

TABLE 3–2   The Military Alphabet

A	Alpha	N	November
B	Bravo	O	Oscar
C	Charlie	P	Papa
D	Delta	Q	Quebec
E	Echo	R	Romeo
F	Foxtrot	S	Sierra
G	Golf	T	Tango
H	Hotel	U	Uniform
I	India	V	Victor
J	Juliet	W	Whiskey
K	Kilo	X	X-Ray
L	Lima	Y	Yankee
M	Mike	Z	Zulu

disaster response including law enforcement, fire service, emergency medical services, the incident command post, other medical facilities, and any other response organization. A persistent issue with external communication is compatibility. It is likely that all of the organizations listed have different communication systems on different frequencies. This would ultimately require several radios stationed in the hospital.

One possible solution is to work with community organizations to decide who in the hospital should talk to whom within the community. For instance, it is essential that the triage area of the hospital and possibly the ED speak directly with the triage area established in the field. Individual ambulances should only contact the hospital triage area if further direction is required concerning their patient. It is important that the radio system used from field triage to hospital triage be the same as from ambulance to either of the triage points. Security personnel in the hospital should be able to speak directly to law enforcement and the fire service for obvious reasons. The incident commander and the command center at the hospital should have the capabilities to speak with all internal and external stations.[1,27,28]

All parties should be trained in how to speak over the radio. Protocols should be established for how and when communication takes place. The same terminology used internally should be used externally. Complex codes commonly used by law enforcement may complicate communication but serve to prevent information sharing with non–law-enforcement personnel. These should never be used within the hospital; however, it may be important to understand what they are speaking about. Incorporating reference lists in key areas of the hospital should be part of the disaster planning. Communication must be clear and concise. Limit what is said over the radio to essentials. It is likely that somebody, including the media, is listening. Premature or unclear information may lead to rumors and worse, panic.

One potential way to meet communication needs is the amateur radio community. Amateur radio operators can assist with communication in the disaster setting. Many operators belong to or have organized local, regional, and national groups to provide service during a disaster. The limitation is that only licensed operators may speak on the radio and they may or may not have any knowledge of medicine or disaster response. This requires an operator and radio at all points that wish to speak to each other. An alternative is to have key individuals in the hospital and community obtain a "no code technician class" license. This level does not require knowledge of Morse code, only a basic understanding of amateur radio operations. This would require an investment in hand-held or base-station radios and it may be difficult to set up workable antennas, but this may be less expensive than other dedicated radio systems. Lastly, the frequencies are public, allowing others to listen and speak. Federal Communications Commission (FCC) rules require them to stay off the frequency when it is being used in an emergency, but these are difficult to enforce during a disaster response.

Mitigation is very complex requiring extensive preplanning and awareness of sources of aid only some of which are mentioned here. It is, however, essential. Personnel who prepare the hospital or institution's disaster plan should be dedicated, knowledgeable personnel from all departments of the hospital. Representatives from each area will contribute specific knowledge—both of how they will be affected by a disaster and how they can contribute to the response.

Surge Capacity

Most hospitals operate at or near capacity all the time. If a unit or wing of the hospital does not use most of the beds, it is combined with another unit. EDs begin the day with full carts and remain that way through most of the next 24 hours. Patient wait times are, at best, hours for treatment. If a disaster occurs, waves of hundreds of victims will present to the hospital in addition to the normal day-to-day patients. The number of victims the hospital can care for beyond the normal day-to-day patient load is the hospital's surge capacity.[1,2,29,30]

Most EDs take increases in census in stride. The Emergency Medical Treatment and Active Labor Act (EMTALA) requires that all patients receive an initial evaluation and stabilization. If the number of patients becomes too high, some EDs will defer ambulance patients to other hospitals in the area; walk-ins are never deferred. During a disaster this is not possible. All local hospitals will be overwhelmed with victims. If there is only one health-care facility in the area, deferring patients is never an option. There are short- and long-term strategies that may help.

If the incident that caused the disaster is relatively small and contained, it may be termed a mass casualty incident (MCI). This can be differentiated from a disaster in that a disaster has mass casualties that overwhelm resources completely whereas MCIs may be smaller and, though they certainly stretch resources almost to breaking, they do not necessitate full disaster plan implementation. The incident is contained and normal day-to-day life for the broad community is restored in less than 24 to 48 hours. An example may be an industrial accident with multiple victims and evacuations of some neighborhoods. The number of victims presenting for decontamination, who are injured, or who

WHY IS IT IMPORTANT To Have Drills?

Drills and exercises allow the hospital and staff to test the disaster plan. To do this effectively, drills must be realistic. If the drill is announced, staff and the community will prepare in advance. Although this will provide some practice, it will not test the actual response. Announced table top exercises or case studies would advance the working knowledge of disaster plans and treatment protocols more so than drills. Drills must be as realistic as possible and include aspects of the community that may be part of the hospital's response plan such as emergency medical services, fire, and law enforcement.

are concerned that they are contaminated or injured may be significant and stretch the system for some time, but it is local and contained. With only a few exceptions, hospital staff operate within their normal scope of practice and patients and victims are treated under normal standards of care. In a disaster, the scope of the incident is beyond local. The whole community and beyond is affected and the incident will not be resolved in a relatively short time.[29,31] The result of Hurricane Katrina, the catastrophic tornadoes in Kansas, or major flooding along the Mississippi and other rivers are examples of disasters.

Short-term strategies to increase the surge capacity of hospitals will increase the hospital's ability to initially meet the needs of either an MCI or disaster. They include:

- **Cancel all elective surgeries and procedures.** The operating rooms and areas where procedures are performed should be held open for treatment of those victims most in need. The space may be used as an alternative treatment area or holding area.[29]
- **Expedite those patients who are scheduled for discharge.** This may be a problem if they are going to be discharged to the area of the MCI or disaster, but if they can be safely discharged, it should be expedited.
- **Transfer step-down patients as the Med/Surg floors open beds.** This allows those patients in intensive care units who can be moved to step-down to be moved.

- **Institute communication protocols between the ED and the floors and units of the hospital.** This allows the ED priority in moving patients to the floors most appropriate to the patient's needs.
- **Institute the disaster or MCI triage systems.** Patients are divided into those who need to be seen immediately, those who can wait, and those who can wait even longer. In a disaster, there may be those who are sent home without definitive treatment or who are allowed to die so that needed resources are used to save others.[2] (See Chapter 2, Triage.)
- **Establish holding areas where those victims and patients who can wait can be kept comfortable.**
- **Establish protocols allowing nurses to decide who needs certain labs, tests, and treatments.** Nurses should be able to order labs, tests, and certain medications and treatments to facilitate treatment when the physician or practitioner is not able to see the patient.
- **Implement protocols that allow social workers and admission personnel to assist in identifying victims and facilitating communication with their families.**
- **Use all extra beds and carts so that patients and victims can be seen in hallways and other makeshift areas.**[29] Although patient privacy is always a concern, saving lives take precedent.
- **Call in extra staff for all areas of the facility.** Extra nurses, physicians, and practitioners will certainly be needed. Just as importantly, admissions personnel, social workers, janitorial and maintenance personnel, aides, food service workers, and others will be needed to meet the needs of the hospital. Establish a disaster call-out procedure to call in extra staff.

These strategies require preplanning and training. It is essential that the institution's disaster plan establish treatment protocols, communication protocols, designate initial treatment and holding areas to be used for various aspects of the response, designate tasks for all hospital personnel, and establish lines of authority. Triggers should be established to implement each phase of the disaster plan. The triggers for these protocols should be specific to the needs presented by the level of disaster. Certain protocols would go into effect for an MCI whereas more extensive treatment and communication protocols would be in effect during a disaster. Some personnel would be called in for an MCI; however, all personnel would be called in for a disaster. Some stable patients may be discharged during an MCI but in a disaster there would be no place to send them. Most importantly, the plan needs to establish when the normal standards of care may be deviated from for treatment of victims and patients. It may be appropriate for victims of an MCI to be treated under the usual standards; it is unrealistic to believe that this will be the case during a disaster[1,2,29] **(see Figs. 3–8 and 3-9).**

Long-term strategies require even more preplanning and will take longer to implement. They include:

- Opening a shuttered or alternative facility. Preplanning for opening a shuttered facility or alternative site is extensive.

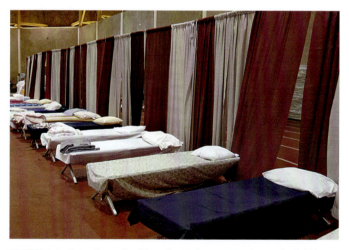

FIGURE 3–8. Baton Rouge, Louisiana, September 3, 2005. Cots at the field house at Louisiana State University await evacuees of Hurricane Katrina. Surge hospitals may be created by opening closed buildings that may be suitable or by converting arenas or other large areas into hospitals. *Photo by Liz Roll.*

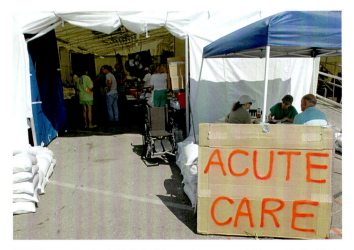

FIGURE 3–9. Waveland, Mississippi, September 11, 2005. A Disaster Medical Assistance Team (DMAT) treats patients in Waveland, Mississippi. DMAT teams help hospitals in disaster areas. *Photo by Mark Wolfe/FEMA.*

Utilities need to be turned on and someone needs to be responsible for the cost—possibly not the owner. Equipment and supplies need to be brought in and organized. These same items will be needed at the traditional facility so these supplies need to be designated specifically for this use.[30]

- Staffing shuttered facilities with food service, janitorial and maintenance services, administrative, security, and others. They will be needed to provide care and meet other concerns.

- Maintaining the shuttered or alternative site during down times to be sure that temperature control, utilities, and building structure remains intact. This may be easy for facilities in regular use but is not always obvious for shuttered facilities. Tents may be helpful but will have limited usefulness in severe heat and cold conditions.

- Using alternative treatment and holding areas such as tents, arenas, warehouses, or empty department stores, or calling for federal response such as DMAT, PERT, and Disaster Mortuary Operations Response Team (DMORT).[25,30]

- Having DMAT, PERT, and DMORT teams that increase surge capacity of an area.[25] They can be stand-alone facilities to provide care for victims and mortuarial services for the deceased. To be activated, the governor must declare a disaster and request their services. They then will take 24 to 48 hours to respond and become functional. They are self-contained units, designed to function completely on their own. They bring and set up their own tents and have all of the needed medical equipment and supplies. Deployment is usually 2 weeks or longer. The DMORT teams after Hurricane Katrina were functional for months after the storm.[26]

Increasing surge capacity is difficult, complex, and most efficient with extensive, realistic preplanning. Long-term solutions in particular require extensive preplanning and may incur expenses the institution is not prepared to meet. Regardless, disasters do happen and when they do waves of hundreds of victims may present to the hospital. Effective planning will make treatment of the victims more effective and efficient and decrease the stress and strain of the staff.

Summarizing the Hospital Disaster Plan

The hospital disaster response plan according to The Joint Commission must be realistic, specific to the needs of the hospital and community, and meet specific guidelines. It must be integrated into the community's response plan. It must establish lines of authority, specifically the hospital-based incident command structure. It must address communication concerns, supplies, community resources, utility concerns, staffing issues, and provide for drills to provide training and test the effectiveness of the plan.[1,4,8,32–34]

1. **Integration With the Community.** The hospital must integrate its disaster plan with that of the broader community. The all-hazards approach mandated by The Joint Commission requires the hospital to examine specific risks the community may encounter and prepare for them. A hospital in a rural area without heavy industry may not require extensive

decontamination equipment; one that is located near chemical industries or along major transportation routes will. The hospital should work with other response organizations to ensure that victim collection and triage is done in a common manner to ensure an effective and efficient response. Resources available to assist the hospital and what the hospital may provide the community should be explored. The hospital may assist in the education of the public and joint grants may be obtained to bolster equipment and training of personnel. The whole community experiences a disaster; the whole community should be involved in planning and response[8,23,34–38] **(see Fig. 3–10).**

2. **Lines of Authority and Responsibility.** The hospital must establish clear lines of authority and structure and integrate these into the community's response. The ICS is adapted to the hospital setting allowing for clear lines of authority and designating areas of responsibility. There is one incident commander (IC). He or she needs to be knowledgeable in

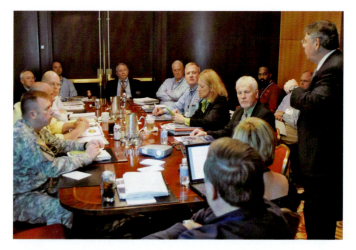

FIGURE 3–10. Atlanta, Georgia, May 4, 2009. A small group breakout session for community disaster planning meeting. Health-care industry, businesses, and government must work together and integrate planning to effectively prepare for a disaster. *Photo by George Armstrong/FEMA.*

disaster response and have the authority to make decisions concerning the utilization of hospital resources and implementation of disaster protocols. He or she needs to have knowledge in administration and medicine. An IC needs to be concerned first for the safety of the hospital and staff, and know that all will be pushed well beyond normal limits. Below the IC are people responsible for each area of the hospital. These areas should have one person with overall control and teams of individuals under them to carry out specific tasks. For instance, there will be one person with authority over the ED. Under that one person will be others designated with authority over triage, specific hold areas, treatment, and other aspects of the ED's response. The hospital's line of authority should be integrated into the community's response. This does not give the community's IC authority over the hospital, but allows for an integrated response with the hospital and the community working together in consensus for an effective and efficient response.[4,26,33,34,36,39–41]

3. **Patient Movement and Treatment Protocols.** Protocols should be developed to ensure efficient treatment and movement of victims during a disaster. Clearly define when disaster protocols will be implemented and what is expected when they are.

   a. What is the role of nursing, nurse practitioners and physician assistants, physicians, security personnel, and other staff? All staff will be called upon to do more than what is normally expected of them, but there are specific concerns for licensed staff. What level of treatment will nursing be allowed to do without receiving an order from a physician or practitioner? What list of medications and under what circumstances will they be allowed to administer on their own? Under what circumstances will some victims be allowed to be discharged without being seen by a physician or practitioner?

   b. What will be expected of practitioners and physician assistants? How will anesthesiologists, surgeons, ED physicians, and other physicians be used beyond their normal role? How will physicians from the community be integrated into the hospital's response? How will volunteer licensed personnel be utilized?

c. Protocols should establish who will be treated first and where treatment will take place. Testing should be limited to only those who absolutely need it. X-rays and CT scans should be limited to those for whom it will affect treatment. Obvious fractures do not require an x-ray during a disaster; neither do minor injuries that would receive a screening x-ray under normal standards. Abdominal and head injuries that may require surgery will require radiological studies even during a disaster. Who decides which victims receive these studies should be clearly established.

d. Patient transport will be altered. Under normal standards, some patients would need to be transported solely by nursing; however, during a disaster it may be performed by aides or untrained personnel. Resources, equipment, supplies, and personnel are limited, if the victim cannot survive testing and treatment, then unfortunately, they will not survive.

e. It is essential to establish clear protocols that will realistically attempt to meet the needs of victims and provide for the safety and protection of the hospital and its staff.[2,17,39,42]

4. **Hospital Disaster Triage and Victim Flow Concerns.** Integrate with the community what disaster triage system will be used and use it. Train all personnel from the hospital and community in its use.

a. Triage in the field should be quick and efficient. Secondary triage in the field and at the hospital is more complex. It decides who of the victims tagged immediate should be treated first and who may need to be reclassified as expectant and cannot be saved.

b. Establish with the community how victims will be transported to the hospital. Who will communicate the victim information to the hospital—the ambulance or, more appropriately, the field triage officer? Will victims be held in the field or in holding areas established at the hospital?

c. Triage and movement of victims is difficult, the hospital and the community must be well integrated.[2,31,39,42]

5. Documentation and victim identification are essential. Under the austere circumstances of a disaster, documentation and victim identification is extremely difficult.
   a. Disaster triage tags should be used in the field and at the hospital. Hospital admission systems should be able to use the number from the tag as the sole identifier; some systems may require letters not alphanumeric or numeric alone.
   b. Documentation is essential. If effective and complete documentation does not occur, the hospital and other emergency services will have little chance of billing for services and recouping some of the costs incurred as part of the disaster response. More importantly, victim care will be compromised. The disaster tag should become part of the victim's permanent chart.
   c. Again, integration with the community for methods, training, and equipment is extremely important.
6. All hospitals must have the ability to decontaminate victims as they present. Even more, hospital ED personnel must be on the alert for victims who are contaminated before they are aware that an incident has occurred.
7. Victims will present "on their own" or be transported by Good Samaritans. They may appear just dirty and may not even be aware that they are contaminated.
8. Decontamination equipment includes showering facilities for victims who can care for themselves and showering facilities for those victims presenting who cannot.
9. Hospital personnel need to be fitted with Level C personal protective equipment and they need to be trained in decontamination and treatment while wearing the protective gear. Level C protection includes Tyvec impervious jumpsuit, neoprene boots and rubber gloves, and a respirator/hood (PAPR hood) or complete face place respirator with hood integrated with the jumpsuit. There should be enough systems available to provide personnel to decontaminate the victims who cannot care for themselves, other personnel to usher ambulatory victims through the decontamination system, and others to provide initial treatment.

10. The decontamination system should be designed to handle the number of victims who may present. In rural areas, it may be expected that there would be few victims, but these victims would still overwhelm most rural EDs.[43] In larger metropolitan areas or areas with large chemical industries, large numbers of victims may present in need.[13]

11. Security is essential during the hospital's disaster preparation and response. Security personnel must control access to the hospital and surrounding area.[44]
    a. Victims should be directed to triage and treatment areas.
    b. Families should be directed to a separate area to wait for information.
    c. The media should be kept in another area where they can be given information yet not have access to sensitive areas.
    d. Security personnel also will be required to keep control of large anxious crowds. Victims will be anxious for treatment but if classified as delayed, they may have to wait a long time. Those victims classified as minor will wait even longer and may be sent home without treatment from a physician or practitioner.[44]
    e. Security personnel must control these situations providing safety for the staff and other victims.[44,45]

12. Drills must be realistic. Most drills are designed to maximize the number of participants so most of the staff is aware and prepared for the drill as it approaches.
    a. Drills should be a surprise and be as realistic as possible without endangering real patients.
    b. Drills should be integrated with the community testing communication protocols, triage procedures, transportation, and other concerns.
    c. Decontamination drills in particular should be realistic to test the time it takes to set up and decontaminate a number of victims.
    d. The Joint Commission requires two drills each year, one may be a table top exercise; the institution should offer more table top exercises and drills designed to test smaller portions of the disaster plan. This would

be effective in keeping staff well trained and test for deficits in the plan without stressing the normal functions of the hospital.[2,8,34,36,38,46]

Summary

Hospital disaster preparation and response is overwhelming. It is the responsibility of health-care institutions to be as prepared as possible to care for as many victims as possible as quickly, efficiently, and professionally as possible. Hospitals and other institutions should be in frequent communication with accrediting and licensing bodies such as The Joint Commission, Public Health, State and federal guidelines for current requirements for disaster planning and response capabilities. This is the responsibility of all of the professional staff at a hospital including nursing. Nursing and APNs will be called upon to perform far beyond their normal scope to effectively manage and treat large numbers of victims and the normal day-to-day patient flow. Establishing plans and protocols to organize and provide guidance to professional staff will result in effective treatment to victims and protection for the staff and the hospital.

REFERENCES

1. Baker MS. Creating order from chaos: part II: tactical planning for mass casualty and disaster response at definitive care facilities. *Military Medicine*. 2007;172(3):237–243.
2. Baker MS. Creating order from chaos: part I: triage, initial care, and tactical considerations in mass casualty and disaster response. *Military Medicine*. 2007;172(3):232–236.
3. Franco C, Toner E, Waldhorn R, Maldin B, O'Toole T, Inglesby TV. Systemic collapse: medical care in the aftermath of Hurricane Katrina. *Biosecurity and Bioterrorism*. 2006;4(2):135–146.
4. Autrey P, Moss J. High-reliability teams and situation awareness: implementing a hospital emergency incident command system. *Journal of Nursing Administration*. 2006;36(2):67–72.
5. Bechtel GA, Hansberry AH, Gray-Brown D. Disaster planning and resource allocation in health services. *Hospital Materiel Management Quarterly*. 2000;22(2):9–17.

6. De Lorenzo RA. Financing hospital disaster preparedness. *Prehospital and Disaster Medicine.* 2007;22(5):436–439.

7. DeJohn P. Hospital supply chain vital part of disaster plan. *Hospital Materials Management.* 2002;27(9):14–15.

8. Bitto A. Say what? Who? Me? Right here in the trenches? Collaborate on what? Seeking common ground in regional all-hazards preparedness training. *Journal of Environmental Health.* 2007;69(6):28–33.

9. Currier M, King DS, Wofford MR, Daniel BJ, Deshazo R. A Katrina experience: lessons learned. *American Journal of Medicine.* 2006;119(11):986–992.

10. Gomersall CD, Loo S, Joynt GM, Taylor BL. Pandemic preparedness. *Current Opinion in Critical Care.* 2007;13(6):742–747.

11. Havlak R, Gorman SE, Adams SA. Challenges associated with creating a pharmaceutical stockpile to respond to a terrorist event. *Clinical Microbiology and Infection.* 2002;8(8):529–533.

12. Hsu EB, Casani JA, Romanosky, A, et al. Are regional hospital pharmacies prepared for public health emergencies? *Biosecurity and Bioterrorism.* 2006;4(3):237–243.

13. Aas P. Future considerations for the medical management of nerve-agent intoxication. *Prehospital and Disaster Medicine.* 2003;18(3):208–216.

14. Banner G. The Rhode Island medical emergency distribution system (MEDS). *Disaster Management & Response: DMR.* 2004;2(2):53–57.

15. Esbitt D. The strategic national stockpile: roles and responsibilities of health care professionals for receiving the stockpile assets. *Disaster Management & Response: DMR.* 2003;1(3):68–70.

16. Bravata DM, Zaric GS, Holty J, et al. Reducing mortality from anthrax bioterrorism: strategies for stockpiling and dispensing medical and pharmaceutical supplies. *Biosecurity and Bioterrorism.* 2006;4(3):244–262.

17. Abdel-Monem T, Bulling D. Liability of professional and volunteer mental health practitioners in the wake of disasters: a framework for further considerations. *Behavioral Sciences & the Law.* 2005;23(4):573–590.

18. Campos-Outcalt D. Disaster medical response: maximizing your effectiveness. *Journal of Family Practice.* 2006;55(2):113–115.

19. Gerardi T. The nurse response emergency database: lessons learned. *Journal of the New York State Nurses Association.* 2006;37(1):16–17.

20. Adams LM. Mental health needs of disaster volunteers: a plea for awareness. *Perspectives in Psychiatric Care.* 2007;43(1):52–54.

21. Amaratunga CA, O'Sullivan TL. In the path of disasters: psychosocial issues for preparedness, response, and recovery. *Prehospital and Disaster Medicine.* 2006;21(3):149–153; discussion 154–155.

22. Fothergill A, Palumbo MV, Rambur B, Reinier K, McIntosh B. The volunteer potential of inactive nurses for disaster preparedness. *Public Health Nursing.* 2005;22(5):414–421.

23. Eyre A, Fertel N, Fisher JM, et al. Disaster coordination and management: summary and action plans. *Prehospital and Disaster Medicine.* 2001;16(1):22–25.

24. French ED, Sole ML, Byers JF. A comparison of nurses' needs/concerns and hospital disaster plans following Florida's Hurricane Floyd. *Journal of Emergency Nursing.* 2002;28(2): 111–117.

25. Cohen V. Organization of a health-system pharmacy team to respond to episodes of terrorism. *American Journal of Health-System Pharmacy.* 2003;60(12):1257–1263.

26. Couig MP, Martinelli A, Lavin RP. The national response plan: health and human services the lead for emergency support function #8. *Disaster Management & Response: DMR.* 2005;3(2): 34–40.

27. Chan TC, Killeen J, Griswold W, Lenert L. Information technology and emergency medical care during disasters. *Academic Emergency Medicine.* 2004. 11(11): 1229-1236.

28. Arisoylu M, Mishra R, Rao RA, Lenert LA. Wireless distribution systems to support medical response to disasters. AMIA Annual Symposium Proceedings/AMIA Symposium. 2005;884.

29. Cotter S. Treatment area considerations for mass casualty incidents. *Emergency Medical Services.* 2006;35(2):48–51.

30. Eastman AL, Rinnert K, Nemeth IR, Fowler RL. Alternate site surge capacity in times of public health disaster maintains trauma center and emergency department integrity: Hurricane Katrina. *Journal of Trauma Injury, Infection, and Critical Care.* 2007;63(2):253–257.

31. Auf der Heide E. The importance of evidence-based disaster planning. [see comment]. *Annals of Emergency Medicine.* 2006;47(1):34–49.

32. Arnold JL. Disaster medicine in the 21st century: future hazards, vulnerabilities, and risk. *Prehospital and Disaster Medicine.* 2002;17(1):3–11.

33. Annelli JF. The national incident management system: a multi-agency approach to emergency response in the United States of America. *Revue Scientifique et Technique.* 2006;25(1):223–231.

34. Lusby LG, Jr. Are you ready to execute your facility's emergency management plans? *Journal of Trauma Nursing*. 2006;13(2):74–77.

35. Ablah E, Nickels D, Hodle A. et al. "Public health investigation": a pilot, multi-county, electronic infectious disease exercise. *American Journal of Infection Control*. 2007;35(6): 382–386.

36. Bender JEM. National incident management system (NIMS) guidelines for hospitals and healthcare systems: designing successful exercises. *Journal of Healthcare Protection Management*. 2007;23(2):41–46.

37. Farmer JC, Carlton PK, Jr. Providing critical care during a disaster: the interface between disaster response agencies and hospitals. *Critical Care Medicine*. 2006;34(3 Suppl):S56–S59.

38. Niska RW, Burt CW. Bioterrorism and mass casualty preparedness in hospitals: United States, 2003. *Advance Data*. 2005;(364):1–14.

39. Born CT, Briggs SM, Ciraulo DL. et al. Disasters and mass casualties: I. General principles of response and management. [see comment]. *Journal of the American Academy of Orthopaedic Surgeons*. 2007;15(7):388–396.

40. Briggs SM. Disaster management teams. *Current Opinion in Critical Care*. 2005;11(6):585–589.

41. Lusby JR, Leonard G. Are you ready to execute your facility's emergency management plans? *Journal of Trauma Nursing*. 2006;13(2):74–77.

42. Farmer JC, Carlton PK Jr. Hospital disaster medical response: aligning everyday requirements with emergency casualty care. *World Hospitals and Health Services*. 2005;41(2):21–24.

43. Furbee PM, Cohen JH, Symth SK, et al. Realities of rural emergency medical services disaster preparedness. *Prehospital and Disaster Medicine*. 2006;21(2 Suppl):64–70.

44. Bullard TB, Strack G, Scharoun K. Emergency department security: a call for reassessment. *Health Care Manager*. 2002;21(1):65–73.

45. Luizzo AJ, Scaglione BJ. Training security officers to recognize the perils of weapons of mass destruction and pandemic flu contaminates. *Journal of Healthcare Protection Management*. 2007;23(2):1–9.

46. Gebbie KM, Valas J, Merrill J, Morse S. Role of exercises and drills in the evaluation of public health in emergency response. *Prehospital and Disaster Medicine*. 2006;21(3):173–182.

Personal Preparedness

Introduction

There are extreme circumstances in which it is impossible to prepare **(see Fig. 4–1).** For instance, living on the coast, remaining behind when told to evacuate, and having about 30 feet of water push through your house trapping you in the attic as your house floats off its foundation is something a person cannot be prepared for. Individuals who have very little typically lose the most and are least able to purchase even those few things needed to be personally prepared. Most people and disasters do not fall into these extremes. Most people are able to take a few steps to ensure survivability of most disasters.

Personal preparedness at its simplest is being physically and mentally prepared to meet basic needs for at least 3 days without outside help. Taking this one step farther, being truly prepared is being able to survive virtually where ever you are for 3 or more days under even the most difficult circumstances.

Personal preparedness and a sense of increased awareness are vitally important to individuals within the health-care system. If individuals become victims and are unable to care for themselves, they are unable to care for others around them. Nurses and other health-care professionals may be unable to effectively respond in the work environment or the field if they are uncertain if their needs and the needs of their families are being met. These significant and appropriate concerns will be distractions and, combined with the environment of the disaster, place the responder and victim in potential jeopardy.

Public health nursing also should work with the general population in educating and facilitating personal and family preparations for disasters. A well-prepared and educated population may sustain less illness and injury related to a disaster. They will have a better understanding of the dangers and potential risks associated with where they live and be prepared to react to threats.

Personal and family preparedness and an increased awareness also should be a part of nursing preparation and continuing education. Nurses have a significant influence on their work environment and their neighborhoods. Their knowledge and efforts to prepare will have an impact on professional and nonprofessional colleagues and to their neighbors.

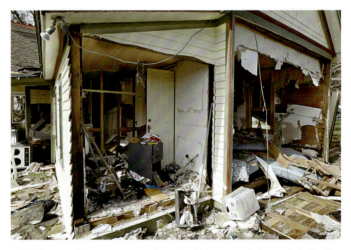

FIGURE 4–1. When a storm surge is 30-feet high or tornado-force winds develop seemingly out of nowhere, there is little chance of surviving in your home. Most disaster events, however, are not that quick or destructive. When survival is possible, the home should be stocked with food, water, and other supplies needed for a minimum of 3 days. When forced to evacuate, it is important to have supplies and important papers in easy access in case of trouble on the road. *Photo by Gene Dailey/American Red Cross.*

Planning

Personal preparedness is an ongoing process of planning and cache needs for yourself and those in your care. As with any planning, begin with a risk assessment. Each person's or family's risk varies depending on what part of the country, type of dwelling and where it is located, and transportation concerns. Ideally, an individual's personal preparedness plan (PPP) should encompass every aspect of a person's life. As with any disaster planning, the limitations of finances and freedoms influence the extent of planning. Personal preparedness plans must be realistic and comprehensive. Developing any preparedness plan first requires a risk assessment. Decide first what the risks are:

- Are there dangers that would require a person or family to be confined to the home for an extended period? Are there dangers that would force a person out of the home quickly and for a significant amount of time?
- Will there be a warning?
- Will the whole structure be a safe haven or will only a part of it be safe?
- What weather affects the area—flooding, tornadoes, hurricanes, major snow storms, or earthquakes? **(See Fig. 4–2.)**
- Do long commutes or other extensive travel place a person or family on the road for a long period of time?
- Is the immediate or extended family and loved ones close by or spread out?
- What are the employment requirements in the event of a disaster? Those who work in the health-care industry will

be expected to report to work as necessary to treat those affected by the disaster.

- What communication options are available such as cell phones, radios, hard wired land lines?
- What needs will there be to contact family members within the area affected by the disaster or those outside the disaster?
- What temperature extremes will need to be prepared for and do they change throughout the year?

Often one question in the risk assessment inspires several more. It is important to not become paralyzed by a task that starts an ongoing process that changes, expands, and contracts as life changes. In the end, decide what the significant risks are and what you can prepare for. Decide when to remain in place and, if given the chance, when you will leave and seek other shelter.

In general individuals and families should be prepared to shelter in place for 3 days without outside assistance. A

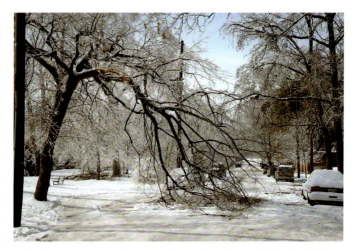

FIGURE 4–2. Severe weather may make roadways impassable forcing victims to be stranded either in their homes or on the road. Food, water, and clothing appropriate for the weather is essential for the home, vehicle, and workplace. *Photo by Daniel Cima/American Red Cross.*

person's home should have enough food, water, medicine, sanitation, and environmental needs for 3 days.[1–4]

Water

Water is essential for personal preparedness. Under normal conditions, most of us need about 2 quarts of water per day. Food preparation, sanitation, and other activities increase this amount. It is recommended that 1 gallon of water per day per person be stored. Store the water unopened in its original container if purchased commercially. Use or cycle the water by the expiration date. If water is stored in reused containers, use clean plastic containers that has not been used for milk or juice. The proteins from these liquids cannot be completely removed and will cause the water to spoil. If the water source is a well or water that is contaminated, filter the water and treat with chlorine bleach, ten drops per gallon. Allow treated water to stand for 30 to 60 minutes before drinking. The best way to decontaminate water is by boiling. Again filter the water and bring to a rolling boil for 1 minute. Allow to cool before drinking. Store water prepared this way only for 6 months. Other sources of water in the home include the hot water tank and pipes. Care should be taken to turn the hot water tank off before draining it. Do not use water from pools or spas. If a shortage of water is anticipated, fill bathtubs, buckets, or sinks with water before the supply is turned off. This water may be used for sanitation purposes **(see Table 4–1).**

Use caution if water needs to be collected from outside the home. Rain water can be safely used as drinking water, whereas water taken from ground sources should be treated first. Use water from as clean a source as possible, with as few particulates as possible, and no floating debris. Filter debris and particulates from the water with a towel or coffee filter. The water them should be treated with 10 drops of household bleach per gallon. The bleach should be 5.25% to 6% hypochlorite and not contain scents or other additives. After treating, the water should have a slight bleach smell, if it does not, retreat with 10 more drops of bleach. As stated previously, water can also

TABLE 4–1	Physical Needs for Survival for 3 Days
Water	Enough drinking water and water for sanitation for 3 days, about 1 gallon per person. Store in sealed containers from the store. Add extra water for pets and others who may be in need.
Food	Enough for 3 days, should be easy to prepare, store well without concerns of spoilage and be nutritious and enjoy able. Should require little or no preparation. Add extra food for pets and others who may be in need.
Clothing	Changes of clothing appropriate for the weather.
First aid and medications	First-aid supplies befitting your level of training. Basic over-the-counter medications for humans and those that may be used for pets, such as aspirin. Prescription medications for at least 3 days.
Miscellaneous	Three days of survival may get boring, materials for entertainment for all members of the household.

be boiled for purification. Restore the oxygen content to the water by pouring it back and forth between clean containers; this will help it to taste better. Water also can be purified using portable camping purification systems. These can filter down to 0.3 microns and remove particles, protozoa, and bacteria. Activated charcoal assists in removing chemicals and improving taste. Water can be distilled by boiling and collecting the vapors. The collected vapors will cool becoming drinkable water. Distilling is the only way saltwater can be made drinkable.[3,4]

Evidence for Practice

Water is more important than food, don't conserve, don't skimp, and have enough. Dehydration lessens the body's ability to respond and affects the ability to think clearly. During a disaster, life and death decisions may have to be made and a quick effective response may be necessary. Dehydration will have deleterious effects on those abilities.

Food is important but not as important as water. You should never ration water but, if necessary, ration food. A 3-day supply of nonperishable food should be kept in the home. This supply should be checked periodically for freshness. Some foods such as wheat, rice, vegetable oils, soybeans, bouillon, and dry pasta may be stored indefinitely. Canned meat, vegetables, fruits, peanut butter, jelly, and juices may be stored for up to 1 year or according to the expiration date on the label. Dried fruit, powdered milk, and powdered potatoes may be stored for 6 months. Food should be kept in sealed air tight containers and discarded if there are any signs of spoilage. Backpacking meals or MREs (Meals Ready to Eat) developed for the military provide other options. Often backpacking meals are dehydrated or need to be prepared with water, which will add to the water needs. MREs are complete meals with heaters that require only a small amount of water to activate the heater. Both last for a very long time before having to be eaten and replaced **(see Fig. 4–3).**

The choice of food also is important. It should be easily prepared or require no preparation. Manual can openers, utensils, and other needs should be included in storage plans. It is important to choose food that you and your family enjoy along with treats. Survival is not always enjoyable. A candy bar may relieve boredom on several levels. Include food for any pets that may be part of your household.

Cooking and heating may be difficult. Use camp stoves or charcoal and propane grills outside and only with adequate ventilation. Canned items may be heated in the can after they have been opened and the label removed. The contents may also be eaten without heating.[3,4]

Clothing and Bedding

Circumstances determine if there is access to all of the clothing and bedding in the home; however, if there is a possibility of limited access or if there is a chance of quick evacuation,

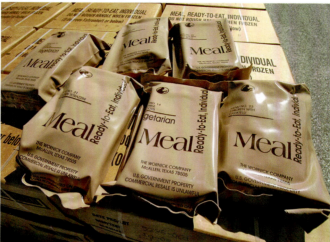

FIGURE 4–3. Woonsocket, Rhode Island, August 9, 2007. Meals Ready to Eat (MREs) are displayed on top of a pallet of cases in position to be placed into the vehicles of "disaster recipients" participating in a hands-on 2-day event hosted by the Rhode Island Emergency Management Agency in conjunction with FEMA. Each case contains a variety of meals and will feed a family of four for 1 day. *FEMA photo by Win Henderson.*

two changes of clothing and bedding should be kept with the supplies. Clothes should be suited to the current weather conditions, but should always include warm clothing. Even in warm weather and warm-weather areas, cool or cold weather can occur.

Sleeping bags suited to the weather should be available for each member of the household. They are rated for specific temperature ranges. A bag rated to –20°F may be perfect for northern states in the winter, but would be inappropriate for the Gulf Coast. Similarly, a bag rated at 35°F would be very inappropriate for a northern winter. Sleeping bags also provide very portable bedding and may be helpful if leaving the house quickly is required. Use padded ground pads for both comfort and warmth when sleeping on the ground or concrete floors.[3,4]

First Aid and Medications

The household first-aid kit should contain basics and items specifically needed for the individual and family:

- Latex gloves
- Sterile dressings with tape and bandages
- Cleansing agents
- Antibiotic ointment
- Eye wash
- Thermometer
- Splinting supplies (Sam splint and Ace wraps)
- Scissors and tweezers

Over-the-counter medications should include:

- Aspirin or nonaspirin pain relievers and to provide fever control appropriate to the age of household members
- Antacids
- Anti-diarrheals
- Benadryl

Also include a 1- to 2-week supply of prescription medications and supplies. Households with special needs should consider additional items. For example, if a member of the household is pregnant, a birthing kit and training to care for mother and child should be considered. People with advanced training such as physicians, nurse practitioners, physician assistants, nurses, and EMS providers may consider adding to the basic kit according to their level of skill and training. Everyone should consider cardiopulmonary resuscitation (CPR) and first-aid training.[3–5]

Miscellaneous Items

Other items include:

- Flash lights with extra batteries; these should be checked periodically
- Tools including a wrench or pliers suitable for turning off utilities and other uses, along with a hammer and screwdrivers

- Camp knife
- Matches (in a waterproof container)
- Small mirror (for signaling and other uses)
- Whistle (to signal for help)
- Moist towelettes
- Garbage bags and buckets (for sanitation, toileting needs, and other uses)
- Items needed for personal hygiene
- Household bleach (may be helpful as a disinfectant and to treat contaminated water)
- Copies of important personal and family papers
- Cash
- Paper and pencil
- Favorite books, games or puzzles for all members of the household[3,4] **(see Table 4–2)**

TABLE 4–2	Checklist of Preparedness Supplies
Water	• Enough for 3 days with a minimum of 1 gallon of water per day per person.
	• Fill sinks and bathtubs with water when possible not for drinking but for sanitation.
	• Unscented chlorine bleach 10 to 16 drops per gallon to purify water, filter particulates before purifying.
	• Camping water purifiers will make most water safe to drink.
	• Never ration water.
Food	• Store enough food for each person for 3 days.
	• Store easily prepared, long-lasting, low-sodium food in a cool, dry place.
	• Store any items needed for preparation with the food.
	• Food should be nutritious and enjoyed by the family.
Clothes and bedding	• Changes of clothing including jackets for 3 days for each person.
	• Sleeping bags appropriate for the climate and sleeping mats for warmth and comfort.

TABLE 4–2 Checklist of Preparedness Supplies—cont'd

First aid	• Latex gloves.
	• Sterile dressings with tape and bandages.
	• Cleansing agents.
	• Antibiotic ointment.
	• Eye wash.
	• Thermometer.
	• Splinting supplies (Sam splint and Ace wraps).
	• Scissors and tweezers.
	Over the counter medications should include:
	• Aspirin or nonaspirin pain relievers and to provide fever control appropriate to the age of household members.
	• Antacids.
	• Anti-diarrheals.
	• Benadryl.
	• Consider other items based on training and medical licensure.
Miscellaneous items	• Flash lights with extra batteries. These should be checked periodically.
	• Tools including a wrench or pliers suitable for turning off utilities and other uses, along with a hammer and screwdrivers.
	• Camp knife.
	• Matches (in a waterproof container).
	• Small mirror (for signaling and other uses).
	• Whistle (to signal for help).
	• Moist towelettes.
	• Garbage bags and buckets (for sanitation, toileting needs, and other uses).
	• Items needed for personal hygiene.
	• Household bleach (may be helpful as a disinfectant and to treat contaminated water).

Continued

TABLE 4–2	Checklist of Preparedness Supplies–cont'd
	• Copies of important personal and family papers.
	• Cash.
	• Paper and pencil.
	• Favorite books, games, or puzzles for all members of the household.[3,4]
Storage	Store all items in a cool, dry, protected place with easy access in an emergency.
Jump bag	Have a duffle bag or backpack with smaller amounts of the items listed above in case quick evacuation is necessary.

Storage

All of these items should be stored together in a cool, dry location. Exactly where they should be stored depends on the risks prone to the area. Areas prone to wind storms would keep the supplies in the basement whereas areas prone to flooding should store items on upper floors. Smaller homes and apartments may have space concerns, but will also have smaller numbers of people to prepare for. If possible, store the supplies near an exit to facilitate loading into vehicles if forced to leave quickly.[3,4]

Travel and the Office

What is necessary for travel is dependent on the part of the country and time of year. Travel of any significant distance by personal vehicle in any part of the country requires a few basics including blankets, food, and water for every person. Every vehicle should have a roadside kit including flares or reflectors, a signal flag, a flashlight or lantern, and a few basic tools.

Day-to-day commuting presents other challenges. Storage of food and water in a vehicle used for daily commutes may be difficult because of weather conditions and temperature extremes. Vehicles parked in the sun in warm climates become extremely hot. Water during the colder parts of the year will freeze. Regardless of these issues, vehicles should be equipped with enough food, water, and supplies for the driver and any passengers to survive if stranded. The supplies needed are similar to those needed in the home.

Stranded at work presents further challenges. For those employed in a health-care facility, food and water may not be a concern. There also may be beds, bedding, and blankets available. Portable generators and other working utilities may provide heat, cooling, and light. However, even if these things are available, they may be in short supply or may have been destroyed by the disaster. Although it may be impractical to have a complete personal preparedness kit at work, it is usually possible to have a change of clothes, basic food items (like protein bars), flash light, and a few other personal needs such as prescription and other medications stored in a locker or office.[3,4]

Communication Concerns

Communication concerns must be addressed as part of the PPP. These concerns fall into two categories: communication with the outside and communication with the family. Communication with the outside monitors the progress of the event, may make the person or family aware of new concerns or the possible need to evacuate, and may be accomplished by portable battery-powered radios or televisions; however, local radio and television stations may not be broadcasting depending on the size of the disaster. Emergency authorities may broadcast important safety instructions over local stations through the emergency broadcast system.

Communication with family may be very difficult. Cell phone signals and land phone lines may work sporadically or not at all. Cable line and phone line outages also would affect Internet access, e-mails, and other computer-based communication. Satellite phones may be functional but they also operate on electricity from either the power grid or battery. If the power is off and batteries are low, even the satellite phone will not be of much use.

WHY IS IT IMPORTANT To Have Good Communication?

Communication issues are extremely important; plan carefully for both receiving information and communicating with others. A battery-operated radio or television may provide information concerning the emergency. This assumes that there will be broadcasts in the area, which may not be true. A weather alert radio will provide emergency broadcasts in more austere circumstances. Keep cell phones charged in an effort to communicate with loved ones. Develop a schedule of when calls will be made and to whom. Consider an amateur radio license to increase chances of reaching family, friends, or help in time of need. Phones may be down so the 911 system may not be operational.

Always keep cell and satellite phones well charged. Establish a plan for when to call; for instance, 20 minutes before the hour in case one or the other party needs to conserve battery power or move to a specific location for signal strength. Decide on someone outside the area to be the person everyone will relay messages through if necessary. Establish a local meeting place if the residence is compromised and have a regular meeting schedule if it is not a place you can go to and stay. Finally, have a meeting place outside the area where everyone can make their way to over time. Clearly establishing a complete communication plan is an essential part of a complete personal preparedness plan.

Attitude and Awareness

All the physical preparedness previously discussed will be of no help to those who panic or believe they are going to die. Those who do not panic and believe they will live stand a much greater chance of survival even without physical needs. Awareness and a positive attitude, not panicking, and making rational decisions is the most important part of a person's personal preparedness plan.

Awareness can be defined as the state of being aware. "Being aware" is a state of being in which one is aware or conscious of both what is happening around and to a person all in relation to their knowledge and past experiences.[6,7] A victim of severe physical trauma may respond to painful stimuli as a part of evaluation and treatment but may not be aware of or conscious of what is going on around them. They respond to the pain by pulling away or tensing their muscles but it is not an integration of the experience with their knowledge or their past. They are not aware.

A person walking along the street who is reading, texting, or so engrossed in thought that they do not recognize the change in the height of the sidewalk, the change in traffic, or that others around them have stopped moving, is not aware. They stumble off the curb and into traffic. They are not conscious of the stimulus or clues around them and therefore are not able to integrate them with their past experiences of walking along a busy street.

Emergency room (ER) providers on a particularly busy night may notice that they have treated multiple patients with a possible diagnosis of Guillain-Barré syndrome. In their minds, they consider a list of differential diagnoses including botulism. They may even question the patients concerning a common food source. Finding none, being quite busy (not an excuse, just a fact), and with the difficulty of diagnosing botulism versus Guillain-Barré and other neurological syndromes and diseases, the provider may not realize that these patients may be the victims of a purposeful release of aerosolized botulism toxin. The providers are certainly aware. One cannot work effectively in the ER without a high degree of awareness, but because of a possible lack of knowledge concerning aerosolized botulism toxin, distraction by other seemingly more critical patients, or lack of experience (no one, as of this writing, has cared for an incidence of mass contamination by aerosolized botulism toxin), the provider is unaware of this possible scenario and the victims may not receive initial essential and appropriate treatment. A terrorist attack would go unnoticed longer than it should.

Being aware is a skill that can be developed both professionally and personally. David Diaz in his book, *Tracking: Signs of Man, Signs of Hope*, recounts his experience as an Army tracker in Korea using subtle changes in the environment left by a terrorist squad to track them until intercepted and finally stopping them. The trackers were aware of small changes left on the ground by boots as the terrorists walked. They were aware of how the changes aged, which provided clues as to how far away the terrorists were. The trackers interpreted the information left where the terrorist rested or camped, providing information on how many terrorists there were, what their training level was, and if there were any civilians within the group. They were aware of safety and security, dealing with booby traps left behind, and knowing when they were close to the terrorists so as to not become victims themselves. The trackers were hyperaware of their surroundings; seeing and cataloging turned pebbles, bruised leaves, scuffs, and human discard; then using their knowledge and experience to know where the terrorists were and what they were doing. They succeeded in intercepting the group and stopping a biological attack[8] **(see Fig. 4–4).**

Similarly, Joel Harding recounts an incident of tracking a criminal well trained in the art of avoidance through a wooded area along the United States northwestern border. The criminal had successfully avoided well-trained police dogs. Harding again used subtle changes left behind on the ground, stones, and logs to track the criminal. Being able to tell how close the criminal was, he was able to take appropriate measures for his safety and apprehend the criminal.[9]

At this writing, there is a gentle breeze blowing through about seven different types of trees with about five different types of birds (either by sight or sound) flying around and several small squirrels running through the tree tops. It

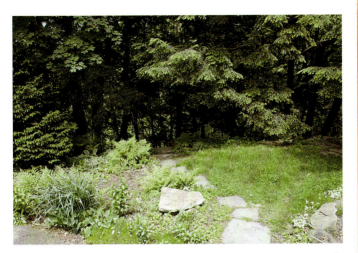

FIGURE 4–4. Increasing day-to-day awareness of the world may protect an individual from assault, terrorist attacks, or natural disasters both large and small. It has the added benefit of increasing an individual's enjoyment of the surrounding world. *Photo by Michael Beach.*

is warm with moisture from last night's rain in the air. There is traffic noise from a nearby highway, insects buzzing, and noise from a heat pump compressor. The wind gently rustles the leaves and wind chimes occasionally strike a note. There are multiple plants, flowers, ferns, and shrubs. The sky is cloudy but bright and the light plays off the moist leaves as they move with the wind. There are multiple butterflies of varying hues in the trees and around the flowers. The squirrels are noisily chirping and debris from their play and from the local woodpecker falls to the ground. These things and thousands of other stimuli would escape someone who only allowed themselves to be aware of whatever project they had on their mind (such as writing this book) as they sat in the conglomerate that is a neighborhood backyard.

Being aware allows people to enjoy their surroundings more fully; it also allows the individual to be safer. Combining an increased awareness of our surroundings and what we know is a "normal experience" in our daily lives, we know when something is missing or is amiss. We would notice a person stepping out in front of us on the side walk and the person walking quickly up to us from behind. We would know that there is no one else around us. Even if we have never experienced being robbed or attacked before, experience would tell us that this is not within our "normal experience." Even if we are wrong about the intentions of the two people (an impending attack), the changes we make in how and where we walk will make little difference except to possibly save a life.

This awareness also applies to multiple presentation of illnesses, such as the flu, out of their normal season or with similar unusual symptoms and should at least raise concerns for health-care providers that this may not be a normal circumstance. Pandemics and epidemics may begin with presentations like this. A few dust-covered patients presenting to the ER may well be simply dirty from a particularly dirty job or they may be the first wave of victims of a chemical spill or dirty bomb. If those victims have injuries that require immediate treatment and they are rushed into a bed without asking some very important questions, then the ER and those treating the victims are now contaminated and further care of other patients and victims is compromised. It is essential that health-care providers be aware of the many varied possibilities that could present from an intentional or unintentional chemical, biological, nuclear, or explosive event. Health-care providers need to be hyperaware

WHY IS IT IMPORTANT To Practice Awareness?

Awareness of what is going on around you will increase chances of survival during a disaster and throughout daily life. Being aware of what is normal will allow awareness of what is abnormal and if that is a danger. During a disaster, threats remain from those with ill or illegal intent. Others are simply in need and may be understandably anxious or panicy. A steady state of awareness will help to differentiate threats from those who are simply in need of help and pose no threat. Increasing awareness increases safety; it also increases enjoyment of life.

of the subtleties of patient presentation, the signs and symptoms of the patients, and complexities of differential diagnosis that may include varied and rarely seen diseases. A common mantra for health-care providers is that they are the first line of defense for the beginnings of pandemics and of terrorist acts. Without the proper knowledge and being conscious of the possibility of disastrous events, we will not be able to compensate for our general lack of experience in recognizing and treating such rarely seen events; events such as pandemic outbreaks of flu, or intentional releases of the plague, botulism, anthrax, and worse.

Alert and Awareness Systems

After September 11, 2001 the federal government through the Department of Homeland Security (HS) developed a color-coded alert system to be used nationwide. The system uses green, blue, yellow, orange, and red with green indicating low risk of terrorist attack, blue indicating guarded, yellow indicates elevated, orange indicates high, and red indicates a severe risk of attack. At this writing, the current threat level is elevated or yellow. The instructions on the HS Web site state that "there is no credible, specific intelligence suggesting an imminent threat to the homeland at this time." The site also states that the threat is high or orange for all domestic and international flights (see Table 4–3).

The system was placed into effect on March 11, 2002 and was initiated at yellow. It was raised to orange near the anniversary of the 9/11 attacks. It was raised from yellow to orange on February 7, 2003, for possible al-Qaida attacks and remained there for 20 days. Ten days later it was again raised to orange in anticipation of attacks coinciding with the invasion of Iraq; it remained elevated for about 1 month. It was raised again about 1 month later for about 10 days. The level was raised one last time in 2003 near the holiday season extending into 2004. A close examination of these and other changes in the alert level reveals relatively rare instances where the level is raised to that of severe and never lowered

TABLE 4–3 Homeland Security Color-Coded Risk System

Green/Low	Indicates low risk of terrorist attack.
Blue/Guarded	Indicates an intermediate level of concern for terrorist attack.
Yellow/Elevated	Indicates a concern for a terrorist attack but no actionable information.
Orange/High	Indicates a high level of concern without actionable information.
Red/Severe	Indicates specific actionable data concerning a terrorist attack.

Source: Homeland Security. Preparedness and Response. 2008. Available at: http://www.dhs.gov/xprepresp/. Accessed August 8, 2008.

past elevated. Raising the alert level is complex and may have a significant economic impact, particularly on the travel and tourism industries. This impact may be tempered by a lack of awareness of these changes by the general public. A system that remains at the elevated, high, or severe levels for extended periods of time may begin to lose its impact. Lowering the level during periods when there is evidence that may indicate an elevated or higher level of concern could also create problems, particularly if an incident were to occur.

The Homeland Security Advisory System consists of three public parts: Homeland Security Threat Advisories, Homeland Security Information Bulletins, and the Color-coded Threat Level Systems. The Homeland Security Threat Advisories are designed to contain "actionable information about an incident involving, or a threat targeting, critical national networks or infrastructures or key assets." This may include new procedures to improve security or a change in readiness, protective actions or response. They are targeted to federal, state, and local governments, as well as some in the private sector and international partners.[10]

Homeland Security Information Bulletins are similar but do "not meet the timeliness, specificity, or significance of threshold" of the threat advisories. They may include reports, statistics, reporting guidelines, or requests for information. These target the same government, private sectors, and international partners as the threat advisories.

The Color-coded Threat Level System is designed for and targeted to both public officials and the general public. It is expected that the public would take appropriate protective measures to "reduce the likelihood or impact of an attack."[10]

As of this writing, the Department of Homeland Security has announced that it will be reviewing the color-coded alert system currently used in the United States. Although somewhat effective when first established, confusion remains concerning what the various levels mean and how they are changed. Confusion also remains concerning appropriate citizen and business response to the levels and when the status changes. Visit the Homeland Security Web site to remain updated on changes and appropriate response.

The Color-coded Threat System has had two opposite effects on society. Raising and lowering the threat level and/or leaving it at the "yellow/elevated" level and "orange/high" for air travel without other specific information or discussion may have numbed the general public to any significant threat. At the same time, the effect of raising the threat level on those who do pay attention may have a significant impact on the economy and personal freedoms. People may shop or travel less and the increase in security certainly may cause increased inconvenience and restrictions on personal freedoms. Examples of these changes from the past include: family and friends no longer being allowed to accompany travelers to the gate at most airports and other than very small amounts of very specific fluids, in very specific containers, you are no longer allowed to have liquids in carry-on luggage. Although these may be small inconveniences and may be necessary, in early commercial aviation no one was screened for weapons, though they were carried at the time and people were permitted to smoke not only in the airport, but in flight. It can be argued that these changes are good and very necessary; al-Qaeda was not operating in the 1930s and 1940s; liquid bombs were not suspected before August, 2006; and, of course, we now know the dangers of smoking, but it should at least give pause to note that with each increase in security we may be better protected but we also are a little less free.

Perhaps most disturbing is the numbness of the general population. In general, people seem to be most concerned about terrorist attacks or disasters after they have occurred. The more distant, both in time and physical distance, people are from an event, the less they believe it will happen to them. Anecdotally, people seem to respond that it may be possible for an event to happen to them but they do not believe it will. When disasters occur, people seem to expect that they will still be taken care of by the local ambulance service; fire department; hospital; or city, county, state, or federal government. People believe a safety net is always there to catch them when they fall. In a disaster, there are no safety nets.

Lieutenant Colonel Jeff Cooper, a World War II and Korean War veteran, began an educational facility near Paulden, Arizona, for fire arms training. Cooper developed his own color-code system. This system does not concern the threat level of the country or area you live in; it concerns the threat level around an individual. The system consists of four conditions; white, yellow, orange, and red. With condition white, people are oblivious to their surroundings. They are preoccupied with something not related to the environment around them. People who live in condition white are not aware of either the good or the bad around them. They are not aware of the changes from the normal that may be occurring around them, they cannot call upon any knowledge, skills, or experiences to help them and guide their actions and decisions. Being unaware, these people are victims before an event happens—be it large scale or personal.[11]

Condition yellow is a general state of alertness. The person is involved in normal activities with normal surroundings and nothing of concern to focus on. The person is, however, aware. They know what fits into the "normal world" around them and are aware of what is not normal.

What is not normal may or may not be bad, it just is not what is regularly encountered and, therefore, deserves greater scrutiny. Whatever is out of place is neither good nor bad, neither a threat nor safe, until it has been assessed. If it is benign, condition yellow continues. If a threat is realized, the person proceeds to condition orange.[11]

In condition orange, people have targeted something or someone who they believe is a threat. Clues associated with the situation are assessed, such as the demeanor and body language of the person or persons of concern. The details of the bag or baggage left in a place it should not be and people who may have been seen with it. Subtle details are noticed that may increase the item's, the person's, or event's level of suspicion. If correctly assessed as a threatening situation, a person's level of awareness advances to condition red. If the threat dissolves, the level moves back to condition yellow.[11]

It is important to continue to be aware of everything in the surroundings as one moves through this process and not focus completely on what has been identified as the threat. What is under suspicion may not be the threat. There may be something wrong but the source may not be what has been identified. The person's knowledge, experience, and awareness has indicated a concern and by narrowing your focus too much, the actual threat may be missed.[11]

With condition red, the threat has been identified and the person is in a state of readiness to act. A planned response has been devised and a trigger has been identified that will cause the person to act. The plan may be to leave the area, call law enforcement, alert others to the threat, act in self-defense, or run. The trigger may be aggressive behavior from an individual or group, smoke or fire, offensive or irritating odors, anything that indicates the threat has escalated and action is needed. The fact that a plan has been developed decreases the time it takes a person to respond to danger. Going through the stages of increased awareness, assessing the situation, developing a plan and trigger enables a person to respond quickly and appropriately. If the trigger point is never reacted, the person simply scales down to condition orange or yellow.[11]

Col. Cooper originally designed this system to deal with threats to personal safety from individuals with criminal intent. However, the conditions and levels of alertness are easily adapted to and interchangeable with awareness in any aspect of life. The same alertness that would save one from being attacked or assaulted would alert one to impending disaster both man-made and natural. Obviously impending severe weather should propel a person from yellow to orange and red with a set plan and trigger to implement it and thereby protect them from possible injury. A truck driving through and stopping in an area where it should may move a person to orange. When the driver gets out and walks away nervously, or worse, runs away leaving the truck unattended, condition red should be considered causing the person to run, upwind and uphill if possible. If nothing happens, laugh and realize that if something did happen, the person, you, would still be alive[11] **(see Table 4–4).**

This system is extremely adaptable to health care, particularly the ER. Health-care providers in the ER are always at condition yellow with occasional moves to orange. Providers are always alert to the needs and concerns of their patients.

TABLE 4–4	Cooper's Color-Coded Awareness System
White	A state of being unaware of anything happening around you.
Yellow	A state of being aware of what is happening around you. You are comfortable with nothing to cause alarm.
Orange	A state of being aware that something is out of the ordinary around you. Something is wrong and you begin to become hyperaware.
Red	Something is wrong, you are hyperaware, you may be in danger. You have isolated the concern, developed a plan to deal with the situation, and are waiting for the trigger to put the plan in action. If the danger dissipates, you move back to orange or yellow.

Source: Givens T. States of Awareness, the Cooper Color Codes. 2004; Available at: http://www.teddytactical.com/ SharpenBladeArticle/4_States%20of%20Awareness.htm.

They are aware of the levels of activity, the number of patients, and what kinds of illnesses have been presenting. Patients or events may propel the provider to a condition orange with swift actions and protocols dealing with the concern. Occasionally they are propelled to condition red. When several (or one, depending on the size of the ER) major traumas, cardiac arrest, or severe respiratory distress present, immediately pre-arranged plans take effect and the "threat" or event is dealt with appropriately and as efficiently as possible under the circumstances. A large number of patients presenting with the same set of symptoms may represent the first wave of victims from a chemical spill and should propel the providers in the ER from yellow to orange and red, recognizing the threat/event and taking steps to institute plans for decontamination and treatment.

Summary

Awareness is an attitude, a healthy state of mind allowing people to enjoy the good around them and protecting them from the bad. It is not a state of paranoia in which danger is looked for where it is not. It is a state in which both the dangers and the good are recognized and are dealt with or enjoy as appropriate.

Nurses and other health-care providers must be in a constant state of awareness and preparation. This allows them the ability to respond appropriately to the dangers around them in a disaster and in their everyday life. It has the added benefit of limiting burnout through an appreciation of the good, beautiful, and noble around them.

People also should be aware of alert systems such as the HS color-coded system. The HS color-coded system alerts us to threats on a local, regional, or national level. It is based on credible evidence obtained at the various levels of law enforcement and government. The use of this system has affected all aspects of our life in some way, though we may have become numb to the concerns it may raise. Although this is often ignored, it does make providers aware of credible threats. On a personal level, people need to be alert to changes in the world around them both as a matter of protection and enjoyment. Actions taken by the HS system are broad and have significant effects on people's lives.

Awareness as nurses and health-care providers allows them to be better clinicians. They are aware of the broad range of unusual and rare illnesses terrorists may inflict on patients. They become better equipped to respond quickly and effectively to man-made and natural events that may overwhelm by calling for additional recourses and personnel and by instituting the institution's disaster plan early.

On a personal level, being more aware protects people from potential threats by enabling them to act with predetermined plans set off by an established trigger. It allows a person to act and not be oblivious to dangers and be taken unaware. Just as important, being aware allows people to appreciate the sights, sounds, smells, textures, and feelings of what is around us. In general, it is quite enjoyable.

REFERENCES

1. United States Geological Survey. Earthquake Hazards Program. Available at: http://earthquake.usgs.gov/regional/nca/1906/18april/index.php. Accessed March 14, 2007.

2. Board on Natural Disasters. Mitigation emerges as major strategy for reducing losses caused by natural disasters. *Science*. 1999; 284:1943–1947.

3. American Red Cross. Prepare at Home. 2008. Available at: http://www.redcross.org/general/0,1082,0_91_4440,00.html. Accessed October 5, 2008.

4. Hamilton, MG, Lundy PM. Medical countermeasures to WMDs: defense research for civilian and military use. *Toxicology*. 2007;233(1–3):8–12.

5. Hsu EB, Thomas T, Bass EB, Whyne D, Kelen GD, Green GB. Healthcare worker competencies for disaster training. *BMC Medical Education*. 2006;6(19).

6. Yorks L, Sharoff L. An extended epistemology for fostering transformative learning in holistic nursing education and practice. *Holistic Nursing Practice*. 2001;6(1):21–29.

7. Trapp P. Engaging the body and mind with the spirit of learning to promote critical thinking. *Journal of Continuing Education in Nursing*. 2005; 36(2):73–76.

8. Diaz D. *Signs of Man, Signs of Hope.* 2005, Guilford, CT: The Globe Pequot Press. 244.
9. Hardin J. *Tracker.* Self published. 2004;432.
10. Homeland Security. Preparedness and Response. 2008. Available at: http://www.dhs.gov/xprepresp/. Accessed August 8, 2008.
11. Givens T. States of Awareness, the Cooper Color Codes. 2004; Available at: http://www.teddytactical.com/SharpenBladeArticle/4_States%20of%20Awareness.htm.

Violent Weather

5

Introduction

Severe weather and other natural disasters are significant factors in disaster planning virtually anywhere in the world. In the United States, the East and Gulf Coasts contend with hurricanes; the North with cold and snow; the Central Plains and southern states with tornados, or severe storms and flooding; on the West Coast, earthquakes; and several parts of the country contend with drought; each bringing its own share of concerns **(see Fig. 5–1).** Trauma, disease, and infection increase as a result of each of these conditions. Populations are displaced and individuals devastated. Preplanning by governments, institutions, and individuals is necessary to mitigate the effects of, respond to, and recover from severe weather. This chapter cannot cover all types of severe weather or their result. The health-care institution should be guided by its risk assessment and an "all hazards" approach to developing a disaster plan.

In the United States, the history of efforts to mitigate the effects of severe weather begins with the advent of the National Weather Service in 1870 by the federal government. At that time, the prevailing attitude was to build structures in an effort to prevent damage from severe weather such as flooding. In the beginning, efforts to predict severe weather were largely unsuccessful, but they have improved significantly. At one time, structures such as dams, levies, and reservoirs were somewhat successful but have become less so now owing to population growth, financial constraints, and other concerns. More recent efforts have included moving populations away from areas at risk such as islands, coastlines, and flood plains or by forcing populations who remain to cover the risk to their crops or dwellings through private or government-backed insurance. Devastating weather, such as flooding along the Mississippi River and other waterways or hurricanes along the Gulf Coast and Florida, has caused the private sector and local,

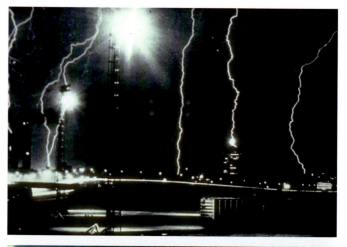

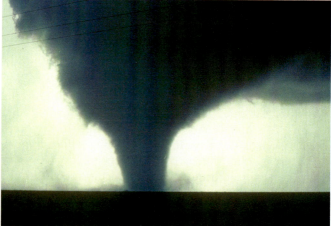

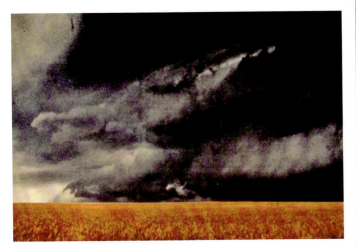

FIGURE 5–1. Disasters are devastating to the natural and man-made environment. FEMA provides federal aid and assistance to those who have been affected by all types of disasters. *Photos courtesy of FEMA/NOAA News.*

WHY IS IT IMPORTANT   To Heed the National Weather Service?

The National Weather Service, which has become the National Oceanic and Atmospheric Administration (NOAA), was first established to survey the coasts of the United States. It now provides a wide variety of services including daily weather forecasts and a system of warnings and watches to help people prepare for severe weather. The system of watches and warnings provide as much time as possible to prepare for severe weather. Ignoring them could cost lives.

state, and federal governments enormous losses in capital, property, productivity, and human life[1] (see Fig. 5–2).

Efforts by the federal government through agencies such as the Federal Emergency Management Agency (FEMA) and Homeland Security have experienced mixed reviews. Significant resources have been mobilized to respond to natural disasters in the form of evacuations, medical personnel, supplies, food, water, ice, and temporary housing. FEMA Search and Rescue (SAR) teams respond immediately to find and aid victims in the immediate area of a natural disaster. Disaster

Medical Assistance Teams (DMAT), Disaster Mortuary Operational Response Teams (DMORT), and Disaster Veterinary Assistance Teams (DVAT) are mobilized after a state of emergency has been declared by the state's governor and a request is made to the federal government. The federal response may last for weeks or months; in some instances, years.[2]

It can be difficult to mobilize large amounts of aid on short notice. Stockpiling of supplies at multiple sites can be expensive. Large purchases of supplies, housing, and other needs at the last minute may be even more expensive. Weather may be something we can anticipate, but responding to its devastation is difficult. Financial restraints combined with limitations of government response and personal freedoms make adequate preparation and response nearly impossible even when we know from both history and immediate warnings that devastation is imminent.

Nursing is an important part of this response. Nurses are a part of the local health-care response and the teams

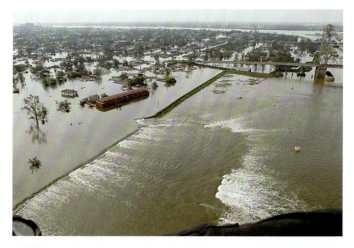

FIGURE 5–2. New Orleans, Louisiana, August 30, 2005. Aerial photograph of the break in the levee in the 9th ward. Neighborhoods throughout the area remain flooded as a result of Hurricane Katrina. *Photo courtesy of Jocelyn Augustino/FEMA.*

brought in by the federal response. Public health nursing works to prepare areas for disasters and responses through local health departments and agencies such as the American Red Cross. Because of this role, nursing educators must provide in-depth instruction covering disaster preparedness and response as it applies to nursing. Advanced practice nurses must know how to apply their knowledge and skills to the sometimes unique circumstances created by disasters. Health-care providers should remember that besides those made victim by the disaster, there will always be the normal day-to-day patients in need. All will need to be cared for.

Tornadoes

Tornadoes are extremely violent, unpredictable storms that can cause severe devastation (see Fig. 5–3). They generate the most violent winds of any storms on earth. Although they may form almost anywhere, the terrain and weather patterns in the United States make it more susceptible to tornadic activity than any place else. Tornadoes are cause by warm moist air moving in from the south being overlaid by cool, dry air from the north. Thunderstorms form along the line where these two air masses meet, known as the "dry line." Some of these storms become super cells with tops reaching 35,000 to 45,000 feet. The interaction between these weather patterns is thought to create funnel clouds. When these funnel clouds touch the ground, they are termed tornadoes.[1,3,4]

Tornados can exhibit sustained winds of more than 300 miles per hour and may travel very unpredictable paths. Although they move in straight lines, their contact with the ground and the damage they cause jumps along that line. They are classified by the Fujita-Pearson scale, F0 through F5, with F5 being the most destructive. This was initially based on damage caused by the storms; it is now based on wind speed. The vast majority of tornadoes are F0 and F1 with only about 1% classified as F4 and F5; however, the majority of the damage is done by these few

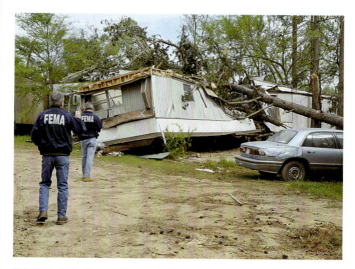

FIGURE 5–3. De Queen, Arkansas, April 16, 2009. Two FEMA Preliminary Damage Assessment officers approach one of the more than 25 mobile homes destroyed by a tornado at Gardner's Mobile Home Park in De Queen on April 9. One of five tornadoes that were documented in western Arkansas struck in Sevier County that evening. *FEMA Photo by Win Henderson.*

WHY IS IT IMPORTANT   To Know About Tornadoes?

Tornadoes travel in a linear fashion causing straight narrow lanes of damage. Most of the damage from tornadoes comes from F4 and F5 tornadoes, which account for only 1% of the total number of tornadoes in a year. These storms are extremely dangerous and cause serious loss of life and property damage. If a tornado approaches, go to the basement. If that is not possible, hide under blankets or a mattress in the interior of the house. If traveling, seek shelter in a substantial building or lie in a ditch. If in a mobile home, get out and seek stronger shelter.

high intensity storms. Whole communities have been completely destroyed by storms of this size. The formation and path of a tornado is somewhat unpredictable, about 60% will occur from noon to sunset. The other 21% and 19% occur between sunset and midnight and midnight to noon, respectively. Tornadoes are most common in the central United States. In

Texas, Oklahoma, and southern Kansas, they are most active in the spring. Frequency then shifts with the season to include the northern central states including northern Kansas, Nebraska, South and North Dakota. Shifting weather patterns may also shift areas and seasons related to the frequency and activity of tornadoes[1,3,4] **(see Table 5–1).**

In May, 1999 a tornado with winds of 316 mph passed through Oklahoma City causing 45 deaths and 637 known injuries, 140 patients were hospitalized, 15,000 structures were damaged, and 10,000 homes were rendered uninhabitable. In 1986, a storm in Pennsylvania caused 91 deaths, 800 injuries, and left 3000 people homeless. A tornado in Illinois in 1990 caused power outages and loss of other basic utilities to more than 65,000 homes and businesses for an extended period of time. The cost in lives from these brief storms is tremendous; the economic cost can also be devastating.[3]

Preparing for a tornado is made difficult because of the unpredictability of the event; therefore, during tornado season, it is important to be aware of tornado warnings and watches. The National Weather Service is responsible for issuing warnings and watches during threatening weather. A **watch** is defined as conditions that are right for the formation of a tornado or other severe weather. A **warning** indicates that a tornado, or other severe weather, has been

TABLE 5–1   Tornado Classification, Wind Speed, and Number of Incidents in 2008

CLASSIFICATION	WIND SPEED MPH	NUMBER OF TORNADOES
F0	40–72	987
F1	73–112	498
F2	113–157	146
F3	158–206	49
F4	207–260	9
F5	261–318	1
Total tornadoes in 2008		1690

sighted either visually or through radar. The Weather Service has deployed Next Generation Radar throughout the United States, which has made predicting tornado activity more precise; at times providing up to 20 minutes of warning.[1,5]

It should be assumed that there will be significant debris scattered throughout the area after a tornado. Roadways will be blocked making access to victims difficult. Power outages and access concerns should be considered when establishing victim triage and collection points and providing transportation of victims to hospitals and other treatment centers. Communication blackouts may occur. Destruction will be in several linear areas. These lines of destruction may be relatively narrow, only up to several hundred yards wide but may be miles long. The destruction will be extensive and there may be lingering danger from storms, flooding, downed power lines, and debris. Structural damage will be extensive and may pose additional danger to survivors and rescuers.[1,3,4]

Common Injuries Related to Tornadoes

The most common injuries related to tornadoes are soft-tissue injuries such as the following:[3]

- Contusions, lacerations, abrasions, and puncture wounds. These wounds will be heavily contaminated with soil and debris. Many of the lacerations will have concomitant contusions. These soft-tissue injuries are common among rescuers as well as victims.
- Fractures are the second most common injury reported. Of these, open fractures are very common.
- Blunt trauma to the head, chest, and abdomen are the least common injuries resulting from a tornado.
  Admission rates for tornado victims run around 25%.
  Wound treatment involves the following:
- Delayed closure due to significant contamination.
- Antibiotic treatment is recommended to cover aerobic gram-negative species such as *Escherichia coli*, *Klebsiella*, *Serratia*, *Proteus*, and *Pseudomonas*, which are common along with Staphylococcus and Streptococcus.

- Tetanus prophylaxis should be provided.
- Puncture wounds should be well irrigated with saline and 1% povidone-iodine/Betadine and left to close by third intention.

Preparation

Preparation and response to tornadoes involves the following:

- Having a well-defined hospital disaster plan that is well integrated with the local community.[2,6]
- The disaster plan should include a well-thought-out and realistic evacuation plan. This must include how patients will be evacuated from the building, where they will be evacuated to, and increased staffing needs to carry out the plan.[2]
- The hospital disaster plan must include input and involvement from all of the professional staff. Nursing, respiratory, building services, and security must be included with administration and medical staff.[7]
- Integrating all of the local hospitals with Emergency Medical Services to decide where victims should be taken and alternatives established if infrastructure damage prevents transport to the most appropriate hospital. For instance, it may not be possible to transport all severely injured trauma victims to the designated trauma center. Preplanning will help to avoid confusion during the incident.[2,8]
- Damage from tornadoes is sporadic and damage to infrastructures may not be extensive. In spite of this, health-care institutions should be prepared to care for potentially significant increases in patients, particularly in the emergency department for 96 hours without outside aid.
- Being aware of shelter during those times when a tornado is possible **(see Fig. 5–4).**
- People must be aware of tornado warnings and watches as they are announced. In the open, they should seek hard shelter quickly.
- If unable to find hard shelter, they should lay down in a low lying ditch. They should not seek shelter under highway overpasses; these become funnels, concentrating the wind.

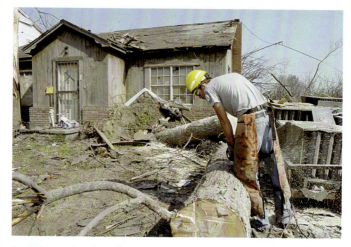

FIGURE 5–4. Caruthersville, Missouri, April 13, 2006. An Ameri Corps volunteer is using a chain saw to cut up a fallen tree and will then haul the debris away. Traumatic injuries caused by the storm and the clean up are common. A tornado hit the town on April 2, 2006. *Photo by Patsy Lynch/FEMA.*

- If driving, park the vehicle and seek shelter in a building or low lying ditch. In a home, the basement, away from windows and sheltered under mattresses, blankets, or pillows is recommended.
- If there is no basement, shelter in an interior room away from windows and doors.
- Mobile homes are the most dangerous shelter during a tornado. Winds as little as 50 mph can cause a mobile home to become airborne. Any mobile homes or mobile home parks should have hard shelters or other protective structures nearby.

Hurricanes

Tornadoes are relatively small localized storms. Hurricanes are large storms that form over open water causing significant devastation when they reach land **(see Fig. 5–5)**. Hurricanes form over the Atlantic Ocean, Gulf of Mexico, or the eastern Pacific Ocean. In the western Pacific and Indian

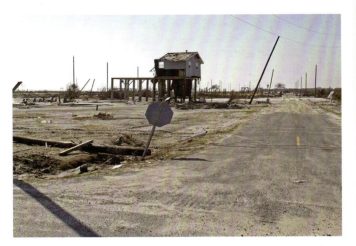

FIGURE 5–5. Johnson Bayou, Louisiana, November 16, 2005. This community at Johnson Bayou was almost totally leveled by the tidal surge and high winds of Hurricane Rita. Hurricane Rita left many people homeless and as of December 20, 2005 FEMA has taken 2,530,657 registrations from Hurricanes Rita and Katrina. *Photo by Marvin Nauman/FEMA.*

Oceans, they are known as typhoons. Hurricanes and typhoons have their beginnings as east to west atmospheric flows over sub-Saharan Africa affecting North America and Central America and from the Gulf of Mexico affecting the western Pacific. These waves meet moisture over the oceans and form tropical waves. The tropical waves that form off the coast of Africa can be felt as far away as Florida. It is not well understood why one tropical wave develops into a hurricane and another does not. It is known that two conditions need to exist. One, there needs to be a positive transfer of energy from warm ocean or gulf waters to the storm system and, two, the absence of upper atmosphere tropospheric wind shear. There are several other factors that also influence the development of tropical waves into storm systems.[1,3,4]

Tropical waves first develop into tropical depressions. Tropical depressions are the beginnings of organized circular storms with sustained winds of 38 mph or less. The next phase is a tropical storm. Tropical storms are organized systems of strong thunderstorms in circular bands with sustained winds of 39 to

75 mph. As the storm increases in intensity, it becomes classified as a hurricane when sustained winds surpass 75 mph. The circular structure of the hurricane creates a central core or eye, which is clear and calm. Winds form a circular wall around this eye. The low atmospheric pressure in the center of the storm creates a "storm surge" as the ocean rises in response. The storm surge is often 50 to 100 miles in diameter and 10 to 20 feet in height with additional storm waves on the surface. A storm surge also increases in height when the off-shore region is shallow. When the storm surge strikes land at the same time as high tide, it is known as storm tide and may be particularly devastating. Storm surges, at high tide from shallow off-shore waters create the highest most devastating conditions. It is important to note that the storm surge and the accompanying storm waves are the most devastating aspect of a hurricane.[1,3,4]

Hurricanes are classified according to Saffir-Simpsom intensity categories. They are classified as Category 1 through 5 depending on the central pressure of the eye, the sustained winds, and the height of the storm surge. Category 1 hurricanes have a central pressure of greater than or equal to 980 mbar, 74 to 95 mph sustained winds and a storm surge of 3.28 to 6.56 ft. In contrast, Category 5 hurricanes have central pressures of less than 920 mbar, winds of 155 mph, and a storm surge of greater than 18.04 ft. Storm waves are on top of the storm surge. **Hurricane warnings** are issued when a hurricane is within 24 to 48 hours of landfall. A **Hurricane watch** is issued when the hurricane will reach an area within 24 hours[1,3] **(see Table 5–2).**

WHY IS IT IMPORTANT To Comply With Evacuation Orders?

The most devastating aspect of a hurricane is the storm surge and the storm waves accompanying them. This storm surge violently raises the level of water from a few feet to as high as 30 feet causing significant damage. The storm surge from Katrina traveled miles inland because of its extreme height. Structures may be swept away or destroyed endangering anyone who may have sought shelter. If an area is told to evacuate, there is no reason strong enough to force a civilian to stay.

TABLE 5–2 Hurricane Classification, Pressure, Wind Speed, and Storm Surge

HURRICANE CLASSIFICATION	BAROMETRIC PRESSURE IN MBAR	SUSTAINED WIND SPEED (MPH)	STORM SURGE HEIGHT (FEET)
1	>980	74–95	3.28–6.56
2	965–979	96–110	6.56–8.2
3	945–964	111–130	8.2–13.12
4	920–944	131–155	13.2–18.04
5	<920	>155	>18.04

Hurricanes have caused widespread damage and death, more so before current advances that accurately predict where and when a hurricane will make landfall. It is estimated that in the past century 74,800 deaths have occurred as a result of hurricanes. Widespread wind, flooding, tornadoes, storm surge, and waves all contribute to a wide area of damage, injury, and deaths. Injury and death can be minimized if those at risk heed evacuation warnings.[1,3,4]

Common Injuries Related to Hurricanes

Injuries associated with hurricanes are varied. They occur from windblown debris and collapsing structures causing trauma and crush injuries or from flooding.[3,9,10]

- Significant flooding may cause drowning to those affected by the storm surge or the heavy rains associated with hurricanes.
- Lacerations, both for victims and rescuers, are by far the dominant injury associated with hurricanes.
- A number of other injuries and illness occur related to contamination or vector-borne disease. Mosquitoes, rodents, snakes, and other wild or domesticated animals will be displaced and have increased contact with humans. Shelter for local inhabitants will be disrupted, people, food, and water supplies will have increased contact with insects and animals.

Rabies should be considered for any animal bite if the animal cannot be isolated. Animal bites should always be treated for infection.[9]

- Only diseases endemic to the area will spread but there may be a spike in the number of people affected. For instance; rats may become a problem after a disaster. Plague, spread by fleas associated with rats will only spread if plague is a known disease to the area before the disaster. Mosquitoes will not spread malaria in an area where malaria is not endemic, such as the United States; however, West Nile virus or St. Louis encephalitis may become public health issues in those areas where outbreaks have occurred before the disaster.

- Potable water may be difficult to find because water supplies may become contaminated by seawater, industrial wastes, chemicals, or sewage. This is particularly a concern for private wells, though municipal water supplies also will be affected. Pediatric poisonings may occur related to inadequate storage of hazardous material such as chlorine bleach, insecticides, or other household chemicals. There does not seem to be any increase in cases of tetanus after flooding or hurricanes, but normal tetanus prophylaxis protocols should be followed.[9]

Damage from hurricanes can be extensive and may involve large areas. Some of the preparations that health-care institutions make for major storms such as tornadoes are the same for hurricanes but because hurricanes can cause widespread damage, some aspects of the plans take on more meaning.[4]

Preparation and response to hurricanes include the following:

- Having a well-defined hospital disaster plan that is well integrated with the local community and state and federal plans.

Evidence for Practice

Most of the injuries in floods and hurricanes are soft-tissue injuries and lacerations. All wounds are heavily contaminated. Prophylactic antibiotic therapy should always be considered and tetanus antitoxin administered if necessary.

In addition to concerns expressed in Chapter 3, hospitals need to prepare for the long-term recovery needs of the institution and the community.[2,6]

- The disaster plan should include a well-thought-out and realistic evacuation plan. This must include how patients will be evacuated both from the building and potentially from the area, where they will be evacuated to, transportation concerns, and increased staffing needs to carry out the plan.[2]
- The hospital disaster plan must include input and involvement from all professional staff. Nursing, respiratory, building services, and security must be included with administration and medical staff. It must address the long-term needs of staff and patients for extended periods of time without outside aid.[2,7]
- Integrating all of the local hospitals with Emergency Medical Services to decide where victims should be taken and alternatives established if infrastructure damage prevents transport to the most appropriate hospital. For instance; it may not be possible to transport all severely injured trauma victims to the designated trauma center. Preplanning will help to avoid confusion during the incident.[8]
- If the community is under an evacuation order, the general population should evacuate. Plans by the community should include transportation for those without private means and shelter outside of the immediate area. The hospital may not be able to evacuate so preplanning may help to meet the needs of staff and patients. However, expect the unexpected and prepare for austere circumstances.

Flooding

Flooding is the most common disaster known. Flooding is a common occurrence related to hurricanes; it is also a very common disaster in its own right **(see Fig. 5–6).** Most religions have a catastrophic flood story as part of their literature and most countries or cultures have been significantly affected

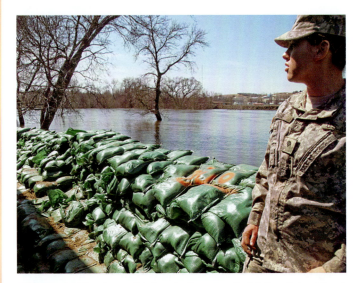

FIGURE 5–6. Valley City, North Dakota, April 14, 2009. North Dakota National Guard, Shayla Longie helps to protect homes along the Sheyenne River by running a 125 gal/min pump behind a dike made of sand bags. The river crested at a historic level of 22 feet. The old record was 19 feet. *Photo by Michael Rieger/FEMA.*

by flooding at times throughout their history. In spite of efforts to mitigate the effects and degree of flooding though structures such as levies, locks, and dams, flooding remains a significant concern today.[1,3]

Societies throughout history have accepted flooding as a trade off for using land around rivers and coasts. Low-lying, fertile land with a plentiful water source is excellent for farming. Waterways, be they rivers or coast lines, are excellent means of transportation. Cities and towns started along these waterways have become significant metropolitan areas. As populations have increased, the number of people living and working in these flood prone areas has increased significantly. Buildings and paving of the land to create roads and parking lots is a direct result of population growth; it also decreases the land available to absorb rainfall. This runoff directly increases the level of water in rivers and streams and contributes to flooding during heavy rains.[1,3]

River systems are made up of larger rivers fed by smaller tributaries along its course. Significant rainfall along the course of the river or its tributaries may cause the river to rise above flood stage in either the area of the rain or downstream from the rain. Flash floods occur when extremely heavy rains occur in terrain above small steams and tributaries, or when earthen or ice dams along rivers and streams burst causing large amounts of water to rush downstream. One of the most famous flashfloods occurred in 1889 when the earthen dam above Johnstown, Pennsylvania, burst after heavy rains. A 40-foot wall of water descended on the town causing significant damage and loss of life. No warnings were received in town in spite of efforts by those at the dam because the telegraph lines were down. People, houses, and other structures were swept downstream. As debris collected, the structures caught fire from the wood- and coal-burning stoves. Many of those who were trapped died in the fire, which burned for 2 days.

When flooding occurs, all of the populations, farming, and industry along the water way are at risk. Levies have been built to attempt to control the damage caused by floods and these have been successful for the most part, though rivers regularly rise above these levels. There is usually significant warning that a flood is about to occur allowing levies to be reinforced and belongings to be moved to higher ground or floors. In spite of this, flooding causes significant loses of property each year. As with tornadoes and hurricanes, there is significant damage to infrastructure,

ALERT!

Swift water is the most dangerous aspect of floods. As little as 2 inches of swift water will knock people off their feet and 2 feet will cause a vehicle to float. Do not attempt to cross swiftly moving water. If trapped, wait for help to arrive and draw attention to yourself by signaling in any way possible. Swift water rescue is extremely dangerous. Do not attempt it if untrained or ill equipped. Never approach swift water without a personal floatation device (PFD) and always be equipped and dressed to survive if attempting a rescue.

crops, and buildings. The force of floodwaters is far stronger and much more devastating than it appears. As with the storm surge of a hurricane, water will move houses and buildings off of their foundations, and destroy bridges, roads, and railroads[1,3] **(see Fig. 5–7).**

Drowning, related to flooding, generally occurs with flash floods or when people do not heed the warnings concerning high water. Floods exert a tremendous amount of force. With flash floods, particularly when earthen dams fail, the water rises quickly and may take residents by surprise. A few inches of swift water is enough to cause a person to fall and create dangerous circumstances. Two feet of swiftly moving water is enough to cause a motor vehicle to float and be swept off the roadway. Most drowning occurs from motorists not heeding high-water warnings and attempting to drive through swift water. People living in low-lying areas must be aware of and heed warnings issued concerning the potential for flooding, in particular, flash floods.[1,3]

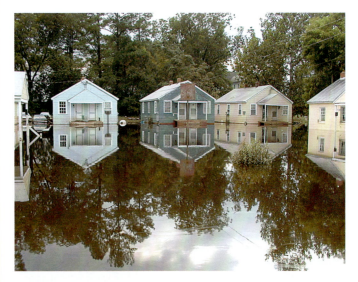

FIGURE 5–7. Franklin, Virginia, September 21, 1999. Flooding left the downtown section of Franklin under 6 feet of water after Hurricane Floyd. As the water has began to recede, as shown by the high-water marks, hazards remained including propane tanks, gas tanks, chemical barrels, and pesticides. *Photo by Liz Roll/FEMA.*

Evidence for Practice

Only those diseases that are endemic to an area will spread after a flood, hurricane, or other disaster. If the area has never had a case of diphtheria, it will not appear just because of the disaster. Those diseases that are endemic to an area and may be exacerbated by sanitation concerns may certainly be of great concern. Planning within the community and hospital should include steps to treat those who contract the disease and prevent its spread.

Common Injuries Related to Flooding

Other injuries related to flooding are similar to those caused by hurricanes.[9] Although there are generally no hurricane strength winds, there may still be significant storm damage related to the weather systems bringing the rain. This damage and debris may make it difficult to find and care for victims. As with hurricanes, the majority of injuries include the following:[3]

- Lacerations and soft-tissue wounds received by both victims and rescuers. These wounds should be considered heavily contaminated.
- Water and food also will be contaminated causing gastritis and gastroenteritis if consumed.[9]
- Vector-borne illnesses may rise.[9]
- Any diseases that are endemic to the area will spread. Diseases not endemic will not be a problem. If cholera is not endemic, it will not be a concern; however, in the United States, West Nile virus and St. Louis encephalopathy may become a significant public health concern.
- Animals displaced by flooding also will be a concern. Wildlife and domesticated animals will have their food and water sources disrupted and will look for replacements. Food stores gathered by survivors should be protected. Interactions between humans and animals may lead to animal bites.[9]
- If rabies is endemic to the area, it should be considered for every bite if the animal cannot be found and isolated.
- Flooding also may cause caskets and bodies in cemeteries to float up from the ground increasing the potential for contamination. DMORT teams spent months after Hurricane

Katrina identifying bodies of victims of the flooding and from caskets found displaced from cemeteries. Bodies of people and animals that perished in the flood will begin to decompose creating more contamination.

- Water-treatment facilities, farms, and industry located along flooded rivers will cause significant contamination concerns. This will affect water sources, both municipal and private. It is important to note that contamination will be a concern even after the water has receded. Soil and groundwater will remain contaminated for some time after the flood.[9]

Preparation and Response to Flooding

- Having a well-defined hospital disaster plan that is well integrated with the local community and state and federal plans. In addition to concerns expressed in Chapter 3, hospitals in potential flood plains need to prepare for the long-term recovery needs of the institution and the community.[2,6]
- Flooding is a process that is usually slow to evolve. Although there are instances of flash flooding that may occur very quickly, large-scale flooding evolves over days and weeks. Health-care institutions should anticipate their needs and the needs of the community before they develop.[2]
- Unless the hospital is located in the flood plain, evacuation may be unlikely. However, flooding may be associated with strong storms and may cause the need for limited evacuation of patients and staff. The evacuation plan should be well-thought-out and realistic. This must include how patients will be evacuated both from the building and potentially from the area, where they will be evacuated to, transportation concerns, and increased staffing needs to carry out the plan.[2]
- The hospital disaster plan must include input and involvement from all professional staff. Nursing, respiratory, building services, and security must be included with administration and medical staff. It must address the long-term needs of staff and patients for extended periods of time without outside aid.[7]

- Integrating all of the local hospitals with Emergency Medical Services to decide where victims should be taken and alternatives established if infrastructure damage prevents transport to the most appropriate hospital. For instance; it may not be possible to transport all severely injured trauma victims to the designated trauma center. Preplanning will help to avoid confusion during the incident.[8]

- If the community is under an evacuation order, the general population should evacuate. Plans by the community should include transportation for those without private means and shelter outside of the immediate area. The hospital may not be able to or may not need to evacuate. Preplanning may help to meet the needs of staff and patients. However, expect the unexpected and prepare for austere circumstances.

Summary

The National Oceanic and Atmospheric Administration was established in 1807 and was the first United States government scientific agency. It was initially charged with surveying the coast of the United States. Since then it has grown to meet the needs of the nation in many ways. Facets of the agency provide daily weather forecasts, track storms, climate changes and their effects across the country. They monitor earthquake activity along the Pacific Rim and provide tsunami warnings to affected coastal areas. They provide tornado, flooding, and hurricane warnings and watches to affected areas and other activities affecting populations and industries. When preparing for severe weather, the most important action that populations at risk can do is to heed those warnings and watches.[1]

A tornado watch may provide 20 minutes or less before the tornado strikes and a tornado warning may be issued much earlier as the conditions develop that are right for their development. In the case of hurricanes, warnings will be issued 48 hours in advance and watches 24. Flood watches also may be issued with 24-hour or longer notice or short notice in the case of flash flooding. Flooding may be forecast days in advance. Warnings are usually issued with significant time to prepare. Each warning should provide enough time for the at-risk population and health-care institutions to prepare.[1]

Nursing and health-care providers should remember that all of the normal concerns and illnesses will continue during a severe weather event. Babies will be born; heart attacks and strokes will occur; the general population will still experience congestive heart failure, urinary tract infections, and pneumonia. Diabetics will go into crisis, children will have ear infections, and mental health patients will have crises. People with special needs will still have those special needs.[11–13] Special diets or tube feedings will have to be given. Those who rely on home health for wound care, medication administration, and other concerns will still require care.[14] Some surgeries may be able to be cancelled but there may be urgent surgeries that cannot be postponed without detriment to the patient. All of the normal day-to-day occurrences will occur during the disaster and in the evacuation centers. Preplanning specifically for both normal needs and for those with special needs is essential to mitigate and prepare for these concerns. Where possible, those with special needs should be identified.[14] If evacuation is necessary, they should be evacuated first to a location prepared to meet their needs.

Evacuations from either the hospital or the community will be difficult and stressful. Preplanning and practice moving patients down stairwells or setting up and using temporary hospitals is important. Early action by the community may help to avoid congested roadways. Adequate personal preparedness will provide food, water, and comfort when none is available in the hospital or on the road. When extreme weather is forecast and the evacuation order is issued for the community, there is no reason to stay and the institution must place all of its preparations into effect. In a battle between man and weather, weather will win.

Shelters are very stressful and difficult. Living in close quarters with strangers on cots set up on a gym floor with common public bathrooms and shared shower facilities are difficult conditions. They are often bright noisy places with little or no privacy. Close quarters also provide excellent conditions to spread common diseases such as the flu or respiratory conditions. Inadequate sanitation will cause gastritis and gastroenteritis and health-care providers must anticipate the need for treatment and possibly isolation.[9,11] Children may have a difficult time understanding the restrictions placed upon them as they share this space. All of this will increase physical and emotional stress significantly. Regardless of these difficulties, evacuation to a shelter, if no other option exists, provides victims with shelter from the extreme weather, a source of food and water, and access to medical care.

Emergency Medical Services and other rescue personnel will be hampered by debris strewn roadways and damaged infrastructure. This will make extrication of victims difficult. Once the storm has passed, medical helicopter transport may be used to extricate some injured or ill victims. Teams on foot may be the only help available to some areas. During flooding, boats may be useful, though this depends on the swiftness of the water. If the water level and force is high enough, highlines, and other technical rescue techniques may be necessary. It is important to note that boat handling during a flood and technical rescue techniques are extremely dangerous and require significant training and expertise.

Extreme weather is devastating though often predictable. Whole communities have been destroyed by hurricanes, tornadoes, and floods. Property damage, economic loss, hardship, illness, and loss of life can be attributed to the effects of severe weather. Populations should heed severe weather warnings and watches issued by the National Weather Service and follow their recommendations. All people should have a personal preparedness plan and supplies to facilitate either evacuation or to provide for their needs if they find themselves trapped. Although it may not be possible or at least likely to survive a 20-foot storm surge and waves without access to high ground and protection from hurricane force winds, or possible to survive winds of 300 mph in a category 5 tornado, most areas will not experience these devastating forces. For the majority of people affected by severe weather, it takes preparation to survive; preparation on the part of local, state, and federal governments, integrated with the medical community and the individual.

REFERENCES

1. National Oceanic and Atmospheric Administration. Available at: http://www.noaa.gov/. 2009 Accessed May 2009.

2. Farmer JC, Carlton PK Jr. Providing critical care during a disaster: the interface between disaster response agencies and hospitals. *Critical Care Medicine.* 2006;34(3 Suppl):S56–S59.

3. Hogan DEB, Burstein JL, eds. *Diaster Medicine.* Philadelphia, PA: Lippincott Williams & Wilkins; 2002, 432.

4. Veenema TG, ed. *Disaster Nursing and Emergency Preparedness for Chemical, Biological, and Radiological Terrorism and Other Hazards.* 2nd. New York, NY: Springer Publishing Company; 2007.

5. Liu S, Quenemoen LE, Malilay J, Noji E, Sinks T, Mendlein J. Assessment of a severe-weather warning system and disaster preparedness, Calhoun County, Alabama, 1994. *American Journal of Public Health.* 1996;86(1):87–89.

6. Pierce JR Jr, Pittard AE, West TA, Richardson JM. Medical response to hurricanes Katrina and Rita: local public health preparedness in action. *Journal of Public Health Management & Practice.* 2007;13(5):441–446.

7. French ED, Sole ML, Byers JF. A comparison of nurses' needs/concerns and hospital disaster plans following Florida's Hurricane Floyd. *Journal of Emergency Nursing,* 2002;28(2):111–117.

8. Einav S, Feigenberg Z, Weissman C, et al. Evacuation priorities in mass casualty terror-related events: implications for contingency planning.[see comment]. *Annals of Surgery.* 2004;239(3):304–310.

9. Ivers LC, Ryan ET. Infectious diseases of severe weather-related and flood-related natural disasters. *Current Opinion in Infectious Diseases.* 2006;19(5):408–414.

10. Ragan P, Schulte J, Nelson S, Jones KT. Mortality surveillance: 2004 to 2005 Florida hurricane-related deaths. *American Journal of Forensic Medicine & Pathology.* 2008;29(2):148–153.

11. Bailey JH, Deshazo RD. Providing healthcare to evacuees in the wake of a natural disaster: opportunities to improve disaster planning. *American Journal of the Medical Sciences.* 2008;336(2):124–127.

12. Kleinpeter MA, Norman LD, Krane KN. Dialysis services in the hurricane-affected areas in 2005: lessons learned. *American Journal of the Medical Sciences.* 2006;332(5):259–263.

13. Lamb KV, O'Brien C, Fenza PJ. Elders at risk during disasters. *Home Healthcare Nurse.* 2008;26(1):30–38; quiz 39–40.

14. Ross KL, Bing CM. Emergency management: expanding the disaster plan. *Home Healthcare Nurse.* 2007;25(6):370–377; quiz 386–387.

Pandemics

6

Introduction

A **pandemic** may be defined as an epidemic outbreak of a disease beyond the local region, usually involving multiple countries. An **epidemic** is an outbreak of an endemic disease beyond normal levels or a widespread outbreak of a new pathogen infection within a geographic area. Both epidemics and pandemics are caused by any outbreak of an infectious disease; noninfectious diseases are never considered as epidemics or pandemics. For instance, cancer, which is not an infectious disease, would not be considered as an epidemic or pandemic though it is widespread. Examples throughout history of either epidemics or pandemics include small pox, plague, viral influenza, cholera, typhus, and measles. Major outbreaks of some of these diseases in the past have killed up to half of the world's population. Outbreaks may be caused by poor sanitation, war, famine, crowded living circumstances, poor hygiene, or chance, as in the case of the mutation of a pathogen such as viral influenza, into a more virulent and infectious agent. These events occur when a disease-causing pathogen is spread throughout a population that has no adequate natural immune defense **(see Fig. 6–1 and Table 6–1).**

Epidemics and pandemics may occur as a result of the reintroduction of a disease to a population or through the mutation of the disease into a new strain for which the population has no natural defense. Small pox caused epidemics and pandemics in the past, but was eradicated decades ago through a rigorous worldwide vaccination program. Should it reoccur, populations worldwide no longer have any acquired immunity,

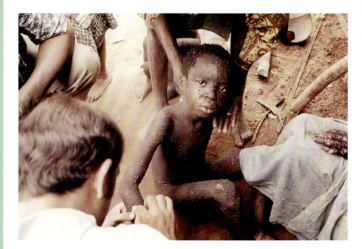

FIGURE 6–1. Photographed in the country of the Republic of Benin, formerly known as Dahomey, sometime during the 1970s worldwide smallpox eradication campaign. This image depicts a small child suffering with a case of smallpox. A health-care provider was providing medical care to the child's maculopapular rash. *Photo compliments of the Centers for Disease Control and Prevention.*

TABLE 6–1   Projected Number of Victims of a Moderate and Severe Viral Pandemic*

STATUS	MODERATE PANDEMIC	SEVERE PANDEMIC
Sick	90 million	90 million
Needing medical attention	45 million	45 million
Needing hospitalization	865,000	9,900,000
ICU	128,000	1,485,000
Ventilator support	64,875	754,000
Deceased	209,000	1,903,000

*Used with permission from the Institute of Medicine.

which would cause rapid, devastating spread of the disease. In today's highly mobile society, where international travel is common, the spread of a new pathological or reintroduced agent could occur quickly; spreading to several areas around the world regardless of the country's socioeconomic development and infrastructure. This chapter describes specifics concerning viral pandemics. The discussions concerning planning and response apply to any potential pandemic.

Nursing and health care need to be particularly concerned about pandemics. These occur regularly throughout history with and without the intervention of mankind. Although countries may work successfully to keep terrorism out and improve living conditions to minimize the spread of some diseases, a pandemic in today's society will cross borders and can affect the most secure and well-prepared country. This means that all countries and populations are susceptible to pandemics.

Pandemics range from very mild diseases that spread from person to person to very serious diseases that spread extremely easily. Populations may be lulled by a mild presentation in the spring and devastated by severe disease the following fall. With a large-scale pandemic, nursing will be called upon to care for those acutely ill, to work in public health, and to educate populations in an effort to properly treat and control the spread of the disease, and in public policy and planning. Nursing may have to adjust practice to increase surge capacity in hospitals and clinics. Nursing educators should prepare undergraduate and practicing nurses for these changes. A prepared workforce will enable an effective response. Nursing administration must supply the support needed to accomplish these tasks and support graduates of educational programs that address these issues in depth.

Pandemic Viral Agents

There are several specific agents with the potential to become a viral pandemic. Viral influenza, including avian flu, swine flu (H1N1), the SARS (Severe Acute Respiratory Syndrome) virus, and the West Nile virus are viruses that currently or have recently caused outbreaks. These outbreaks may or may not follow a seasonal normal flu cycle rising to a peak in late fall, winter, and early spring and waning during the summer months. They may begin in the spring retreat in the summer and become stronger and more virulent in the fall. The viruses may change or develop new strains over time and cause either local epidemics or widespread pandemics. Small pox is a virus that does not exist in the world's population today. Reservoirs do exist in laboratories located in the United States and the former Soviet Union. Should an accidental or intentional release occur the potential for a devastating pandemic is high. Other viral agents or new naturally occurring and mutating viruses may also develop.

Viral Influenza

Influenza is a viral syndrome that causes diseases of both the upper and lower respiratory tract. Seasonally 20,000 to 40,000 people die from influenza despite attempts to predict strains and vaccinate populations at risk. Avian influenza and swine influenza viruses, like all viruses, have shown the ability to combine with genetic material from mammals forming an extremely virulent virus for which their mammalian hosts have no defense. When this occurs, a flu pandemic spreads around the world. In 1918 and 1919, 40 million people died of the Spanish flu. In 1957–1958, 2 million people died of the Hong Kong flu, and in 1968–1969, 1 million people died of the Asian flu.[1–3] The 2004 avian flu outbreak in Southeast Asia and the 2009 swine flu outbreak in Mexico are examples of recent naturally occurring viruses that mutate and become infectious to humans (see Fig. 6–2).

Avian Flu

The World Health Organization (WHO) considers the avian flu virus a significant public health risk as a possible next pandemic. It is caused by the avian influenza A/H5N1 virus and, as of 2007, 258 cases have been documented. Bird-to-human transmission is likely through the fecal–oral route and a 50% mortality rate has been reported. The projected mortality, should regular human-to-human transmission occur, is

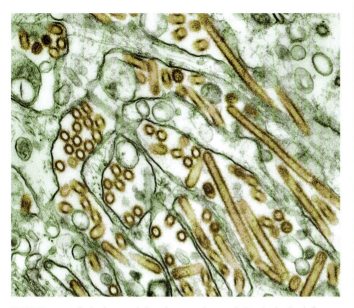

FIGURE 6–2. Colorized transmission electron micrograph (TEM) of Avian influenza A H5N1 viruses (seen in gold) grown in MDCK cells (seen in green). Avian influenza A viruses do not usually infect humans; however, several instances of human infections and outbreaks have been reported since 1997. When infections occur, public health authorities monitor these situations closely. *Photo compliments of the Centers for Disease Control and Prevention.*

estimated at more than 100 million. The disease has the potential to cause significant human and poultry devastation. Avian flu in the human population was first seen in Southeast Asia and migrated to the Middle East, Europe, and former Eastern Bloc countries.[4]

The virus is from the Orthomyxoviridae family. It is single-stranded, negative-sense ribonucleic acid virus. Classification is also based on hemagglutinin and neuraminidase antigens. There are 16 hemagglutinin and nine neuraminidase antigen types. Hemagglutinin mediates the attachment of the virus to the host cell and the neutralization of host antibodies. Neuraminidase cleaves the virus from sites within the host cell creating more sites for replication and spreading the virus through the host. Because of the hemagglutinin type, the avian flu virus has difficulty attaching to a human host. In the past, pigs have been the mediator host allowing the virus to attach to epithelial cells. Viruses then mutate, which may enable human-to-human transmission.[4-7]

The rare human-to-human transmission of avian flu probably first occurred in Thailand from an 11-year-old girl to her mother and aunt. The infection occurred within 3 and 7 days of exposure to the child. All developed fever, progressive respiratory distress, hypoxia, pulmonary consolidations, lymphopenia, thrombocytopenia, and finally shock. The majority of the 18 cases at this writing were related to poultry-to-human transmission. The incubation period appears to be 1 to 8 days with fever, cough, dyspnea, pulmonary infiltrates, and lower respiratory symptoms common upon initial presentation. Other influenza symptoms such as headaches, myalgias, diarrhea, and sore throats also were common. Laboratory results showed lymphopenia, thrombocytopenia, and elevated liver transaminases, although most of these findings were variable from victim to victim. Radiographic results showed bilateral pulmonary infiltrates and manifestations of acute respiratory distress syndrome.[4-7]

Treatment includes immediate isolation. Antivirals with neuraminidase inhibitors such as Oseltamivir or zanamivir may be effective. Amantadine and rimantadine also may be effective. Movement of poultry should be restricted. Culling

Evidence for Practice

Avian flu: The Incubation period is 1 to 8 days. Transmission occurs via fecal-oral or aerosolized. Signs and symptoms include fever, dyspnea, pulmonary infiltrates, lower respiratory illness, headaches, and myalgia. Treatment includes immediate isolation, antivirals with neuraminidase inhibitors such as Oseltamivir or zanamivir may be effective. Amantadine and rimantadine also may be effective. Movement of poultry should also be restricted. Culling of exposed and ill birds should be done with proper disposal of the carcasses. One gram of contaminated manure can infect 1 million birds.

of exposed and ill birds also should be done with proper disposal of the carcasses. Viruses may survive in manure for 3 months and water for 4 days at 22°C and 30 days at 30°C. One gram of contaminated manure can infect 1 million birds. A vaccine was developed and approved by the Food and Drug Administration (FDA) in 2007; however, producing enough vaccine to treat and contain a significant outbreak would be difficult.[4-7]

SARS

A new respiratory disease was reported in southern China in late 2002. By March 2003, it had spread to Hong Kong, and then to Southeast Asia and Toronto, Canada.[8-10] International travel had a significant impact on the spread of the disease from China to Hong Kong and beyond. The WHO declared a global health emergency and mobilized efforts around the world to contain the disease. The early spread of the disease illustrates the ability of a virus to mutate becoming significantly more contagious and severe over a relatively short time. The first cases were a small number of viral pneumonias in Guangdong province in the People's Republic of China. From these cases, each individual's family was affected, but no one else. One of the victims was transferred to a tertiary hospital and finally another hospital for care. The disease quickly spread to 28 hospital staff and the ambulance driver who transferred the patient. A nephrologist who traveled to Hong Kong from Guangdong province while exhibiting symptoms of an upper respiratory illness, stayed in a hotel before being admitted to a hospital in Hong Kong. During this stay, he infected a couple from Toronto, Canada who became ill and spread the disease to health-care workers in Toronto upon their return. The disease became characterized by the high infectivity of health-care workers[9,10] **(see Fig. 6–3).**

The SARS virus is a coronavirus, which is significantly different from other human coronaviruses. There is no evidence of exchange of genetic material with noncoronaviruses. It is thought that the original infection may have come from the consumption of a civet cat, which is considered a delicacy in

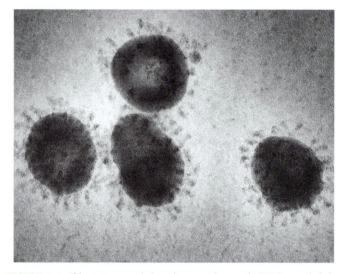

FIGURE 6–3. This 1975 transmission electron micrograph (TEM) revealed the presence of a number of infectious bronchitis virus (IBV) virions, which are *Coronaviridae* family members, and members of the genus *Coronavirus*. IBV is a highly contagious pathogen, that infects poultry of all ages, affecting a number of organ systems including the respiratory and urogenital organs. This is an enveloped virus, which means that its outermost covering is derived from the host cell membrane. The coronavirus derives its name from the fact that under electron microscopic examination, each virion is surrounded by a "corona" or halo. This is caused by the presence of viral spike peplomers emanating from its proteinaceous capsid. One of the most infamous of the coronaviruses is the SARS-CoV, the cause of severe acute respiratory syndrome (SARS). *Photo compliments of the Centers for Disease Control and Prevention.*

southern China. The virus, with the ability to affect the cat, then mutated and developed the ability to infect humans and be transmitted from human to human.[8–11]

Transmission appears to be from aerosolized droplets that are inhaled or come in contact with mucous membranes. The virus is also present in feces. About 25% of victims present with diarrhea, which is another possible source of transmission. It is thought that health-care workers become vulnerable during procedures such as suctioning or intubation and through aerosol, environmental, and fomite spread.[8–10]

Evidence for Practice

SARS: Transmission appears to be from aerosolized droplets that are inhaled or come in contact with mucous membranes. The virus also is present in feces. About 25% of victims present with diarrhea, which is another possible source of transmission. It is thought that health-care workers become vulnerable during procedures such as suctioning or intubation and through aerosol, environmental, and fomite spread.

SARS has an incubation period of 2 to 10 days. Early symptoms include fever, myalgias, and headaches. In addition, some patients present with mild upper respiratory symptoms. After 3 to 7 days, victims begin to develop a dry cough and dyspnea; hypoxia; pulmonary infiltrates follow. Some patients will then develop respiratory failure requiring intubation and ventilation.

Some patients may exhibit a biphasic presentation. Approximately 4 to 7 days after the fever resolves, the victim will develop new infiltrates and worsening respiratory failure. These patients do not do well. Laboratory findings include thrombocytopenia and leucopenia, particularly affecting lymphocytes. Creatine kinase, lactate dehydrogenase, and liver transaminases will be elevated.

Health-care workers are most at risk and should wear an N95 mask.

SARS has an incubation period of 2 to 10 days. Early symptoms include fever, myalgias, and headaches. In addition, some patients present with mild upper respiratory symptoms. After 3 to 7 days, victims begin to develop a dry cough and dyspnea; hypoxia; pulmonary infiltrates follow. Some patients will then develop respiratory failure requiring intubation and ventilation. Some patients may exhibit a biphasic presentation. Approximately 4 to 7 days after the fever resolves, the victim will develop new infiltrates and worsening respiratory failure. These patients do not do well. Laboratory findings include thrombocytopenia and leucopenia, particularly affecting lymphocytes. Creatine kinase, lactate dehydrogenase, and liver transaminases will be elevated. Poorest outcomes were with those patients who presented with advanced age, high peak lactate dehydrogenase, and a high absolute neutrophil count.[8–11]

Early in the development of the pandemic, a clinical trial looked at four treatment options. According to Hawkey[10], the most effective treatment was with high-dose steroids and non-invasive ventilation. Ribavirin, both at that time and today, appears to be ineffective. Today, treatment appears to be the same. Infectious disease experts should also be consulted.[8–10]

West Nile Virus

West Nile virus is caused by a flavivirus that is transmitted from birds to humans through the bite of the culicine mosquito. It was discovered in the blood of a febrile woman in the West Nile region of Uganda in 1937. It first appeared in the United States in 1999, in New York. West Nile virus then spread rapidly across the United States with 9306 cases and 210 deaths by 2003. Most individuals who contract the disease are asymptomatic. Only about 20% of those infected develop flu-like symptoms. Less than 1%, about 1 in 150, develop acute neurogenic disease leading to coma, stupor, paralysis, and/or death[12–14] **(see Fig. 6–4).**

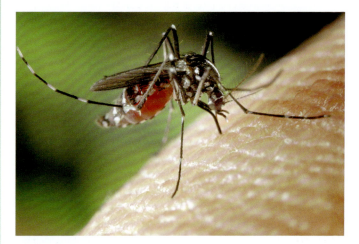

FIGURE 6–4. A blood-engorged female *Aedes albopictus* mosquito feeding on a human host under experimental conditions. The *Aedes albopictus* mosquito, also known as the Asian tiger mosquito, has been found to be a vector of West Nile virus. *Aedes* is a genus of the *Culicine* family of mosquitos. *Photo compliments of the Centers for Disease Control and Prevention.*

Evidence for Practice

West Nile virus: Most victims are asymptomatic. Those who do develop symptoms will present with high fever and chills, lymphadenopathy, backache, anorexia, vomiting, myalgias, and retroorbital eye pain; very few develop encephalopathy. The incubation period is 3 to 14 days. Laboratory tests may show leukocytosis, anemia, thrombocytopenia, and liver enzymes may be elevated. The ELISA IgM will be positive, but also may be positive in patients who have been immunized against other flavivirus. Lumbar puncture analysis may show pleocytosis, increased protein, and normal glucose.

Care is supportive. Ribavirin has not shown to be effective.

Prevention of the spread of the disease is through controlling the spread of mosquitoes in the environment and their bites. Transmission is from a mosquito bite, blood transfusion, organ transplant, by crossing the placental barrier, or through breast milk.

In 2002, it was discovered that the disease was also spread through blood transfusions from asymptomatic blood donors. In response, the FDA recommended screening all blood donations and other sources of transmission, including organs for transplantation. Transplacental and infection through breast milk also should be considered. Titers positive for West Nile virus can be much lower than titers reported for HIV and the hepatitis C virus. Although the quarantine and subsequent removal of infected units of blood may have prevented many cases of West Nile virus, infection through blood transfusion accounted for a few cases. This may be caused by the very low viremia of the disease or other unknown causes.[13,14]

As stated, most victims are asymptomatic. Those who do develop symptoms will present with: high fever and chills, lymphadenopathy, backache, anorexia, vomiting, myalgias, and retroorbital eye pain, very few develop encephalopathy. The incubation period is 3 to 14 days. Laboratory tests may show leukocytosis, anemia, thrombocytopenia, and liver enzymes may be elevated. The ELISA IgM will be positive, but also may be positive in patients who have been immunized against other flaviviruses. Lumbar puncture analysis may show pleocytosis, increased protein, and normal glucose. Care is supportive. Ribavirin has not shown to be effective. Prevention of the spread of the disease is through controlling the spread of mosquitoes in the environment and their bites.[13,14]

Swine Flu H1N1

In the spring of 2009 a new species of the H1N1 virus emerged in Mexico and has infected thousands at this writing. The virus quickly spread to neighboring countries to the north and across the Atlantic Ocean to Europe. Initial cases in the United States, Canada, Scotland, and other countries were diagnosed within days. Mortality rates were significantly higher in Mexico than other parts of the world. This strain is susceptible to current antiviral treatment, which lessens the severity of the disease. In spite of the relatively mild disease, health officials remained concerned that the virus would reemerge during the next flu season with far more morbidity and mortality (**see Fig. 6–5**).

WHY IS IT IMPORTANT **To Be Concerned About Pandemics?**

There are approximately 100,000 intensive care unit (ICU) beds available in the United States. During a severe pandemic, it is projected that we will need 1.4 million ICU beds to care for waves of victims over 1 to 2 years. Approximately 745,000 of these patients will require mechanical ventilation and about 1.9 million will die. A moderate pandemic does not present a much better scenario with 128,000 ICU beds needed and about 65,000 requiring ventilation. Still much more than what is available in the United States. These projections are based on past pandemics and intervening factors such as modern antivirals. Improved medical care and public health policies may decrease the severity of these projections. However, the numbers are so high in comparison to what is available that concern remains.

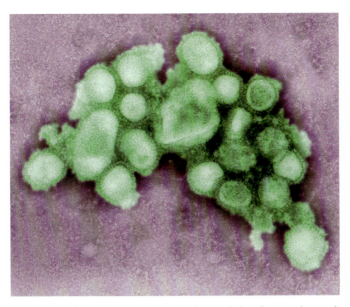

FIGURE 6–5. This colorized negative stained transmission electron micrograph (TEM) depicts some of the ultrastructural morphology of the A/CA/4/09 swine flu virus. What is swine influenza? Swine influenza (swine flu) is a respiratory disease of pigs caused by a type A influenza virus that regularly causes outbreaks of influenza in pigs. Swine flu viruses cause high levels of illness and low death rates in pigs. Swine influenza viruses may circulate among swine throughout the year, but most outbreaks occur during the late fall and winter months similar to outbreaks in humans. The classical swine flu virus (an influenza type A H1N1 virus) was first isolated from a pig in 1930. *Photo compliments of the Centers for Disease Control and Prevention.*

Factors Affecting Emergence of a Viral or Other Pandemic

Viruses mutate through antigenic drift and antigenic shift. **Antigenic drifts** are small changes that occur over time. They are small changes occurring over 1 to 2 years due to a buildup of amino acids as the virus responds to pressures generated by the host such as antibody development. It is because of antigenic drift that the composition of influenza vaccine must change year to year. **Antigenic shift** is a major change in composition caused by the combination of genetic material from two viruses with a change in phenotype or the characteristics of the new virus.[4,6,11] If the new virus is able to infect its host, there would be no natural immunity. Such changes also may lead to efficient human-to-human transmission and changes in the intensity, morbidly, and mortality of the illness.[4–7]

There are multiple factors that affect the likelihood and extent of pandemics, viral and bacterial. These factors fall into four general categories: (1) biological and genetic, (2) the physical environment, (3) ecological concerns, and (4) social and political concerns. The following issues fall into one or more of these categories.[2]

- **Biological Adaptability.** All microbes adapt and mutate. Bacteria adapt, become resistant to antibiotics, and create strains of diseases that are increasingly difficult to treat effectively. Viruses are able to combine with genetic material from other viruses that inhabit or infect the host. The new combination may be more virulent, may be able to be transmitted from human to human, or exhibit other changes. If the avian flu or the swine flu virus combines with genetic material from other viruses and becomes more infectious with increased morbidity and mortality, a new pandemic would occur.[2,9,11,14]

- **Human Susceptibility.** People who are ill, malnourished, elderly, young, or have compromised immune systems are more susceptible to illness in general. Individuals with increased number of social interactions are at increased risk of exposure to a larger number of pathogens. For the West Nile virus, mortality rates are 30% for people older than 70 years of age but less than 1% for those younger. Current projections for a pandemic caused by the avian flu and swine flu indicate that young adults will be more susceptible to the disease.[2,10,14]

- **Climate and Weather.** Climate and weather affect both the human host and the disease. Some virus or bacteria may be more or less virulent depending on temperature. Viruses seasonally affect the population of each hemisphere. Flooding, drought, and other severe weather may cause problems with sanitation, food production, and other issues all of which would either cause or contribute to the spread of disease.[2,4,5,10]

- **Changing Ecosystems.** Changes in the environment have a great affect on the transmission of disease. Waterborne, airborne, food-borne, or vector-borne diseases will be affected by changes to the environment as mankind expands its use of land and water.[2,9–14]

- **Economic Development.** Economic development may have unintended effects on disease. As cities and towns expand, they move closer to animal habitats, which may expose populations to sources of disease. Areas struggling with development, poverty, and overcrowding may be more susceptible to disease.[2,12,14]

- **Human Demographics and Behavior.** The population of the world has increased in its absolute number, urbanization has grown, and large numbers of people live in relatively small areas. There are more people who are immunocompromised from diseases like HIV, cancer, and other chronic diseases. Smoking, alcohol and drug abuse, poor diet, and other behaviors increase susceptibility. The people from these populations are more at risk for the spread of a pandemic because of behavior or simply from their proximity to each other.[2]

- **Technology and Industry.** The use of antibiotics in animal production, large animal farms, and advances in medicine such as blood transfusions and transplants have created new pathways for disease transmission.[2]

- **International Travel.** The rapid daily travel of people and commodities create opportunities for pathogens to travel around the world before symptoms of infection would alert the victims or those around them. Meats, fruits, and vegetables also are transported internationally, creating opportunities for the spread of pathogens.[2,10]

- **Breakdown of Strong Public Health Measures.** The lack of potable water and appropriate hygiene around the world creates opportunities for the spread of disease. Shortages in vaccines, immunization rates that are below target, and increases in nosocomial infections plague developed and undeveloped countries.[2]

- **Poverty and Social Inequality.** The lack of available, affordable health care coupled with the emergence of new diseases throughout the world, increases morbidity and mortality. Questions concerning the ethical distribution of available resources should a pandemic occur have yet to be fully addressed.[2]

- **War and Famine.** The disruption of societies, financial cost, and cost to human life caused by war and famine increases disease morbidity and mortality.[2]

- **Lack of Political Will.** The lack of political will to implement changes that would significantly decrease disease and the microbes that cause them not just in regions where the disease is prevalent but also neighboring regions, plagues not just governments but corporations and individuals.[2]

- **Intent to Harm.** Unfortunately, factions and governments may develop or deploy microbes intentionally to cause harm. Developed nations continue to study bacteria and viruses and hold stockpiles of previously eradicated diseases, such as smallpox, creating the opportunity for an intentional or unintentional leak.[2]

Pandemic Phases

The WHO has developed six phases describing pandemic periods. This may be helpful in establishing trigger points for actions both in preparation and response. There are four periods: the interpandemic period, the pandemic alert period, the pandemic period, and post-pandemic period.[7,15]

- The interpandemic period:
  - Phase 1: No new influenza subtypes have been detected in humans. If a subtype infection is present in animals, the risk of transmission to humans is low.
  - Phase 2: No new influenza subtypes in humans, but there is a circulating animal virus that poses a substantial risk of human disease.
- Pandemic alert period:
  - Phase 3: Human infections with a new subtype but no human-to-human transmission or, at the most, very rare human-to-human transmission from very close contact.
  - Phase 4: Small clusters with limited human-to-human transmission highly localized suggesting that the virus is not well adapted to humans or human-to-human transmission.
  - Phase 5: Larger clusters but human-to-human spread remains local. The virus is more adapted to humans and the risk of a full pandemic is substantial.
- Pandemic period:
  - Phase 6: Increased and sustained transmission in the general population; a pandemic.
- Post-pandemic period
  - Post Peak: Levels of the pandemic have dropped below the peak level in countries with adequate surveillance.
  - Possible New Wave: Levels begin to rise again in countries with adequate surveillance.
  - Post-Pandemic: Levels fall to normal disease levels.

During Phases 1–3, the goal is to strengthen preparations to deal with a possible pandemic, such as stockpiling antibiotics and antivirals. During Phase 4 the efforts should center on containing the new disease and reducing its spread through treatment and vaccination. In Phases 5 and 6 the concern shifts to lessening the affect of the disease on victims and society. During the post-pandemic period, action should focus on lessening the immediate and long-term impact of the disease and prevention of reoccurrence.[15]

Pandemic Planning

Using past viral pandemics as a reference, experts have projected the demands of a viral pandemic on today's health-care system. Scenarios were developed using both the severe Spanish flu pandemic of 1918 and the more moderate viral pandemic of 1957. For both moderate and severe viral outbreaks, the estimated number of sick and those requiring medical care is the same. An estimated one-third of the population in the United States would become ill, approximately 90 million. Approximately 50% of those, about 45 million, would require medical attention. The estimates diverge concerning hospitalizations, intensive care unit (ICU) admissions, patients requiring ventilator support, and deaths. In a moderate viral pandemic, 865,000 would be hospitalized, 128,750 in the ICU with 64,875 requiring ventilator assistance. A severe viral pandemic would require 9,900,000 hospitalizations, 1,485,000 in the ICU with 745,500 on ventilator support. A moderate viral pandemic would cause 209,000 deaths whereas a severe viral pandemic would cause 1,903,000 deaths.[1]

The number of ICU beds in the United States is estimated at 100,000 and they are almost always filled. Ventilators also are usually in short supply. Hospitals generally operate at near capacity with empty beds at a premium. To do otherwise invites financial disaster. Nurses are also projected to be in short supply for many years to come. With only 100,000 ICU beds, in hospitals running near full capacity with a nursing and physician shortage, there will be 865,000 patients beyond our ability to treat. In a severe pandemic, the number of extra patients rises to 9.9 million with 1.4 million requiring admission to the ICU, more than 10 times the number of ICU beds that currently exist.[1]

Although there may be portions of the country or world that are relatively safe from natural or manmade disasters, this scenario is not specific to any one area. In a moderate-to-severe viral pandemic, the severe shortage of hospital beds and treatment facilities would occur wherever the outbreak is most severe. The need for opening shuttered facilities or turning dormitories, indoor athletic facilities, and other indoor facilities into hospitals to increase the surge capacity of the local health-care community will be the only way to treat wave after wave of ill people. Significant preplanning will be required to open these "hospitals" and transport patients from areas affected to those with extra beds. (See Chapter 3.)

Planning involves leadership from community, industry, academic, and government sectors. A cooperative effort to restrict public gatherings, allow employees to work from home whenever possible, close schools and universities if necessary, and restrict travel will help to minimize the local spread of the illness. Local and government health-care officials will need to establish preplans for opening shuttered facilities to care for victims. The public will need to be educated as to when they should seek treatment and where they should report. Trigger points should be established to allow for a phased-in plan to treat victims fairly and avoid restricting freedoms unnecessarily.[1–3,6,7,16–18]

The following outlines what health care, businesses, governments, and colleges or universities may do to minimize the spread and impact of a pandemic.

- Business and Industry
  - Restrict public events.
  - Only essential personnel for business and industry should report to work while others are allowed to work from home if possible or have time off.

WHY IS IT IMPORTANT To Have Public Health Services During a Pandemic?

Public health will need to provide detailed education to the general population concerning when to present for treatment, where to present for treatment, where to go for mass vaccinations or treatment, and how to protect themselves again the spread of the disease. They should work with public officials to develop effective policies to protect the public and prevent panic or other extreme responses. Detailed plans should be made for when and how to close schools, allowing workers to work from home, and restricting public gatherings.

- Assume that more than one-third of the workforce will be unable to present to work as a result of illness, death, or caring for loved ones.
- Government
  - Stockpile and distribute antivirals, antibiotics, and vaccines.
  - Provide funding for opening and staffing emergency hospitals, shuttered facilities, and other sources of care for hundreds of thousands to millions of victims.
  - Restrict public transportation.
  - Close schools allowing students to work from home via computer.
  - Consider restricting travel and commerce, and establishing quarantine areas.
  - Establish who within the government and health care has the authority to order a quarantine.
  - Establish protocols surrounding restrictions including:
    - Use of force to restrict movement in and out of quarantined areas.
    - Legal responsibilities and liabilities of and for the people quarantined.
    - Provisioning those quarantined.
    - Meeting other needs of those quarantined, including health care.
  - Establish a list of essential personnel who must report to work to keep the infrastructure running.
  - Assume that more than one-third of the workforce will not be available related to illness, death, and caring for loved ones.
- Colleges and Universities
  - Set trigger points and protocols to close the college or university.
  - Establish a list of essential personnel who will be required to come to work and train back-up personnel for their positions.
  - Make arrangements for as many employees as possible to work from home or have time off.
  - Allow students who are either too ill to travel and those for whom travel would be unwise to stay on campus.
  - Establish separate living arrangements for well and ill students.

- Establish protocols to provide treatment to ill students in dormitories without hospitalization.
- Each course should be organized so that it could be taught by another instructor or over the Internet.
- Establish protocols for offsite access to faculty and staff computers to facilitate continuity as faculty and staff are forced to work from home.
- Establish protocols for advancement and graduation without physically being present for all or part of a semester or quarter.
- Assume that more than one-third of faculty, staff, and administration will not be able to work from campus or home related to illness, death, or care of loved ones.
- Health Care
  - Educate the public that treatment for influenza needs to begin within the first 48 hours.
  - Preplan for opening shuttered facilities to provide additional hospital beds through:
    - Establishing protocols for opening utilities, cleaning, supplying, and providing equipment and personnel.
    - Educating the public on where to report for treatment.
  - Stockpile essentials including medications such as antivirals, antibiotics, IV fluids, linens, N95 masks, powered air-purifying respirator **(PAPR)** hoods, gowns, gloves, other personal protective equipment (PPE), and supplies.
  - Fit test **all** hospital personnel with N95 masks and consider PAPR hoods for personnel in critical areas.
  - Establish an environment of safety where all personnel wear PPE whenever appropriate regardless of discomfort, inconvenience, or other concerns, including patient contact and comfort.
  - Establish ethical guidelines for the distribution of a vaccine (as it becomes available), hospital space, and medications if they become scarce.
    - Vaccines should be distributed first to emergency medical services; personnel in the emergency department and intensive care areas including physicians, nurse practitioners, physician assistants, nurses; and other staff including environmental staff, social workers, security and other essential support staff.

- Non–health-care workers at high risk also should be vaccinated including those in essential positions, those in close contact with other victims, or those with the comorbidities or risk factors that make them susceptible.
  - The next level would be the same personnel in other hospital-based positions, but in contact with patients with moderate risk of influenza.
  - The third level would again be the same group of hospital personnel but in contact with patients with low risk of influenza.
- Establish an extensive plan concerning hospital and staff safety, distribution points for medicines, triage protocols, canceling elective surgeries and procedures, segregating influenza patients, and limiting patient and staff movement.
  - Establish protocols concerning enforcement of hospital containment measures including who will be allowed into the hospital, where visitors will be allowed to go, and other infection-control measures.
- Assume that more than one-third of the workforce will not be available to work owing to illness, death, or caring for loved ones.

The potential emotional, physical, and economic toll may be significant. In a severe pandemic, it can be expected that approximately one-third of the population will be ill and many of those will die **(see Fig. 6–6)**. Of course less severe pandemics will have significantly less of an impact.

Vaccines

In 2007, the FDA approved a vaccine for the H5N1 avian flu virus; however, until a pandemic occurs because of viral mutation that would increase the virulence and infection rates of the illness, an effective vaccine cannot be assured and mass produced. During late spring 2009, the WHO met to discuss the production of a vaccine for the H1N1 swine flu pandemic. The decision was made to produce a

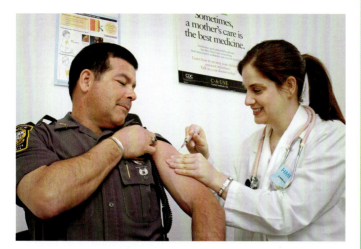

FIGURE 6–6. This 2006 photograph shows a law enforcement officer receiving a vaccination into his left shoulder muscle, which is being administered by a nurse. Health-care workers and other emergency workers should be vaccinated in the event of a severe pandemic. *Photo compliments of the Centers for Disease Control and Prevention.*

WHY IS IT IMPORTANT To Prepare for a Pandemic?

Assume that one-third of the workforce will be sick, or otherwise unavailable to work. The consequences of this is that major portions of industry, public utilities, education, government, and health care will not be available to provide for their normal duties. During a crisis, this can be devastating. In the case of health care, an already strained workforce may be overwhelmed by worker absentees caused by illness.

vaccine for both the H1N1 flu and the projected seasonal flu. The H1N1 vaccine was produced as both an inactivated injectable vaccine and as a nasal weakened live virus vaccine. Although the vaccine was produced using the same techniques and testing as the seasonal vaccine some questions concerning the safety of the vaccine persisted among a few health-care providers and the public. In spite of these concerns, the most common side effect from both the seasonal flu vaccine and the H1N1 vaccine was soreness at the injection site, which resolved after a few hours. Due to efforts to produce both the seasonal and H1N1 vaccines, a limited supply of the H1N1 vaccine was available. A tiered system was developed to ensure those most at risk for complications would receive the vaccine first. The risk factors for complications from the H1N1 virus were again similar to the seasonal flu and included chronic heart, lung, renal, and liver disease; cancer; the immunosuppressed; or women who were pregnant. Obesity (body mass index >30) and morbid obesity (body mass index >40) also appeared to be at increased risk. It was felt that older individuals may have some immunity from previous outbreaks of similar viruses. Those younger than 44 years old were thought to have no immunity to this strain of flu.

The supply of the vaccine was limited as a result of production of both the seasonal and H1N1 vaccine at the same facilities, because of this, smaller-than-expected batches of the H1N1 vaccine were released. In the United States, these were distributed to individual state departments of health for further distribution. Physician or physician groups, local health departments, schools and universities, and clinics then provided the vaccine to the public either through their practices or through mass vaccination clinics. The initial targeted population for the vaccine included pregnant women, persons who live with or care for infants, health care and emergency medical services personnel, individuals ages 6 months to 24 years of age, and individuals 25 to 64 years of age with medical conditions that place them at risk. This was estimated at 159 million in the United States alone. The amount of available vaccine was significantly less than what was projected and its release was much later than expected. Because of this, the initial release targeted pregnant women, some health-care providers, and high-risk children. As production caught up with demand, other individuals were offered the vaccine.

This illustrates the complexity of vaccine development and distribution. Production of the planned H1N1 and seasonal flu vaccine was delayed due to limited manufacturing facilities. Testing was able to be expedited because the H1N1 vaccine was similar to the seasonal vaccine except a different strain of virus, this may or may not be the case in other circumstances. Problems did develop because the virus took longer than expected to grow in the manufacturing process and, in some cases, two injections were required for full immunization, both limiting the amount of available vaccine. Although there were deaths associated with the H1N1 pandemic in 2009, the rates of illness and death were similar to that of the seasonal flu. If this was a severe outbreak of an extremely virulent virus, there would not have been enough vaccine for the large number of potential victims.

In the event of a severe pandemic, there is a targeted group of 500 million people out of a world population of 6.5 billion who should be vaccinated first.[4,5,7]

This list includes the following:

- **Essential Personnel.** These are personnel who are required to keep the major infrastructures open and working effectively such as public and emergency services.
- **Health-care Workers.** These include hospital staff, professional personnel, emergency services, clinic and private practice medical staff.
- **Military and Government Personnel.** This would include essential personnel at all levels of governments and the military.

Others would include:

- Caregivers of those with special needs and the infirmed.
- Those at high risk for death because of age or other comorbidities such as chronic disease.

As a vaccine becomes more available, wider distributions would occur. Significant centers of outbreak would be targeted in an effort to contain the spread of the disease. Herd immunity may begin to limit the outbreak. **Herd immunity** is defined as protection of the uninfected and unvaccinated population because of increasing numbers of the population who have developed immunity either through vaccination or recovery from the disease. This facet of the population cannot become infected and ill and cannot spread the disease to those they come in contact with.

Summary

Pandemics have been caused by many pathogens throughout the centuries. Viruses and bacteria are both susceptible to mutation into new virulent pathogens for which populations have no immunity. Overcrowding, poverty, war, and other conditions can create an environment in which more traditional pathogens such as cholera and typhus could move from a local endemic disease to a broader regional epidemic or pandemic.

Today's fast-paced society commonly travels internationally creating an environment in which new pathogens or new virulent strains of diseases can spread quickly to major population hubs throughout the world before the outbreak is detected at the point of origin. However, as the pace of society has increased, so has the sophistication and effectiveness of health care. The public health disease surveillance and response structures throughout the world are in a position to effectively detect and trace outbreaks of disease. Sophisticated analysis of the pathogens lead to effective treatments and vaccines. Regardless of these advances in health care, societies throughout the world remain at risk for pandemics.

Nursing should prepare to provide public health education and interventions in the form of mass vaccinations and treatments and informing the public about the best practices for preventing spread and obtaining treatment. Hospital disaster planning must include protocols for treating large numbers of victims along with the worried well. Ethics committees should develop guidelines for the allocation of medical supplies and equipment such as ventilators and pharmaceuticals such as vaccines and antivirals. Lastly but of equal importance, quality research is needed to expand our understanding of effective mass-treatment, planning, and prevention.

1. Mason B. *Citizen Engagement in Emergency Planning for a Flu Pandemic: A Summary of the October 23, 2006 Workshop of the Disasters Roundtable*. National Research Council. Washington, DC: The National Academies Press; 2006; 17.

2. Smolinski MS, Hamburg MA, Lederberg, J, eds. *Microbial Threats to Health: The Threat of Pandemic Influenza 2005*. Washington, DC: The National Academies Press; 2005; 40.

3. Committee on Implementation of Antiviral Medication Strategies for an Influenza Pandemic, Antivirals for Pandemic Influenza: Guidance on Developing a Distribution and Dispensing Program. Washington, DC: Institute of Medicine: 2008; 124.

4. Thomas JK, Noppenberger J. Avian influenza: a review. *American Journal of Health-System Pharmacy,*. 2007;64(2):149–165.

5. Bartlett JGM. Planning for Avian influenza. *Annals of Internal Medicine*. 2006;145(2):141–144.

6. Rebmann TP. Preparing for a pandemic influenza. *Journal of Perinatal and Neonatal Nursing*. 2008;22(3):191–202.

7. Scarfone RJM, Alexander S, Coffin SE, et al. Emergency preparedness for pandemic influenza. *Pediatric EMERGENCY*. 2006;22(9):661–668.

8. Denison MR. Severe acute respiratory coronavirus, disease and vaccines: an update. *Journal of Pediatric Infectious Disease*. 2004;23(11):S207–S214.

9. Wang J-T, Chang S-C. Severe acute respiratory syndrome. *Infectious Disease*. 2004;17(2):143–148.

10. Hawkey PM, Bhagani S, Gillespie SH. Severe acute respiratory syndrome (SARS): breath-taking progress. *Journal of Medical Microbiology*. 2003;52(8):609–613.

11. Holmes KV. SARS coronavirus: a new challenge for prevention and therapy. *Journal of Clinical Investigation*. 2003;111(11):1605–1609.

12. Turell MJ, Sardelis MR, Dohm DJ, O'Guinn, ML. Potential North American vectors of West Nile virus. *Annals of the New York Academy of Science*. 2001;951:317–324.

13. McCarthy MM. Newer viral encephalitides. *The Neurologist*. 2003;9(4):189–199.

14. Guharoy R, Gilroy SA, Noviasky JA, Ference J. West Nile virus infection. *American Journal of Health-System Pharmacy*. 2004;61(12):1235–1241.

15. World Health Organization. Pandemic influenza preparedness and response: a WHO guidance document, K Fukuda, H Harmanci, K Park, M Chamberland, E Pluut, TC Niemi, C Vivas, and JK Coninx, Editors. 2009;World Health Organization.

16. Gomersall CD, Loo S, Joyny GM, Taylor B. Pandemic preparedness. *Critical Care.* 2007;13(6):742–747.

17. Glass K, Barnes B. How much would closing schools reduce transmission during an influenza pandemic? *Epidemiology.* 2007;18(5):623–628.

18. DeVille K. Legal preparation and pandemic influenza. *Journal of Public Health Management and Practice.* 2007;13(3):314–317.

Domestic Terrorism: Violence in the Workplace and Schools

Introduction

It is widely accepted that the first mass shooting occurred at the University of Texas, Austin, in 1966 when Charles Whitman climbed to the top of the administration building to the observation deck and began to shoot random civilians. In 1986, Patrick Sherrill walked into the Edmond, Oklahoma post office and shot 14 people sometime after his employment was terminated. In the 3 years before this incident, there were four postal employees killed.[1,2]

Mass shootings in our nation's schools and workplaces seem to be on the rise since the first incident in 1966. Rural schools, large universities, white collar and blue collar areas all seem to be at risk. Reactions seem to vary from severe knee jerk interpretations of "zero tolerance" in which a nail file could cause a student to be suspended or an inappropriate remark without intent may have an employee terminated, to less severe reactions; common to both is less than complete planning.

Schools and workplaces have several similarities with regard to mass shootings. Both have an authority structure that should be involved with preplanning and implementation. Both have authorities that are legally and ethically responsible for the well-being of those in their care either as students or as employees. Both have the near impossible task of interpreting subtle signs and actions of individuals to determine if they are going to act out in a violent manner. Both have a task, as a school to teach or a business to conduct the tasks at hand, that requires maintaining an environment that is comfortable, safe, and without significant disruption. Lastly, both the school's administration and the businesses' executives believe that although shootings happen, they will not happen to them. The problem is that they do happen, which means that it may happen to them.

Some texts have defined mass shootings as an event with more than than five victims from one or more shooters in a 24-hour period. It is important to note that the steps involved with planning, prevention, and reacting to the event may be the same for one shooter and one victim or multiple shooters with multiple victims.[2] In fact, it is reasonable to conclude that appropriate planning and reactions to threats and inappropriate or violent behavior would minimize or prevent loss of life and injury. This chapter will cover the potential for violence in the workplace and in schools and discuss planning and reactions of law enforcement, executives, school personnel, and potential victims. Those perpetrating acts of mass violence in the United States seem to prefer a hand gun, rifle, or shotgun as their tool of violence, however, violence is violence. There are many other potential weapons that should be considered. The release of biological or chemical agents would cause significant harm and injury. Something as readily available as gasoline or other flammable agents in containers with rags as fuses would cause tremendous injury, death, and panic. If these were exploded in a manner effectively blocking exits in a building with many occupants, the death toll could be extensive. In light of this, the terms "workplace or school mass violence" will be used in the place of mass shootings.

Nursing and health-care professionals should be aware of the threat of violence in the home, workplace, and schools. School nurses in particular will be called upon to evaluate threats from those rare students who may be prone to violence. Workplace violence toward nursing is of great concern. Nurses working in the emergency department, psychiatric nursing, and corrections may be at particular risk but nurses working in any environment may come in contact with angry, delusional, or violent patients who pose a threat. This chapter speaks directly to the workplace in general and schools, but the analysis is applicable to any public environment.

Workplace Mass Violence

Workplace mass violence differs from school shootings in that victims and perpetrators are usually adults. This affects some of the planning and reactions. Adults, particularly in the workplace, have certain rights and cannot be controlled the same way as children. Adults may, depending on the state, be permitted to carry weapons either concealed or in the open. Business owners may enact rules that mandate or limit certain behaviors but there are limits involving personal freedoms that must be considered.[1]

Workplace mass violence occurs for several reasons. It may be the result of a disgruntled employee or the result of domestic violence that follows an employee to work. It may be completely random or be related to terrorism. In some cases such as disgruntled employees or domestic violence, there may be ways to prevent the event from escalating to physical violence; in other cases such as random shootings or terrorism, there may only be planning to enable better ways to react. Simply not allowing weapons in the workplace or removing problem employees will not prevent violence. The former employee may simply return and criminals or those who are intent on doing harm will by nature not follow rules concerning weapons. If they are intent on causing harm, they will use whatever tool is at their disposal to inflict death and injury.[1,3,4]

Most workplace violence does not comprise large mass events. Most work place violence involves simple assault, sexual harassment, intimidation and bullying, stalking and other "lesser" crimes. Most of these are not reported to company

WHY IS IT IMPORTANT To Remain Vigilant?

Those who are intent on doing harm will by nature not follow rules concerning weapons. They follow very few rules in general. If they are intent on causing harm, they will use whatever tool is at their disposal to inflict death and injury. Most workplace violence is not of the "mass shooting" nature, but takes the form of smaller crimes. The environment in which nursing often works may be prone to this type of violence. Steps should be taken to realistically protect all employees.

officials, few are reported to the police. In some instances, it is considered a part of the normal environment as it is in the case of many health-care providers, especially nurses.[1,3–5]

Classification of Workplace Violence

The Federal Bureau of Investigation (FBI) classifies workplace violence or mass violence in four ways[1]:

- Type 1 involves violence committed by someone not connected to the institution, such as violence committed during a robbery or other random act.
- Type 2 involves violence committed by customers or students; someone who is served by the institution.
- Type 3 is violence committed against officers or employees by fellow employees or former employees.
- Type 4 involves violence perpetrated by someone who does not work at the institution but has a connection to another employee such as instances of stalking or domestic violence following an employee to work.

Each type has specific measures that can be taken to minimize risk **(see Table 7–1).**

With Type 1 violence, employers can take specific measures to increase basic security for the business and its employees. Specific training for employees diminishes the chances perpetrators have of successfully injuring, killing, or committing other violence against the organization and its employees. These criminals do not have specific connections with either the organization or the employees. Their actions may not be completely random but are based on the possibility of successfully causing mayhem or stealing from the organization. Well thought out security measures may encourage the criminal to attack a less secure location. Conversely, an organization without plans and security may be inviting attack.[1]

The same issues apply to terrorist activities. Part of an organization's risk assessment should be a realistic evaluation of the potential for terrorist attack. Large financial organizations, chemical or biological manufacturing companies, nuclear storage or waste disposal, hospitals and research facilities, and small

TABLE 7–1   Types of Violence and Basic Actions To Be Taken Before Violence Is Committed

TYPE	DEFINITION	WHAT TO DO
Type 1	Violence committed by someone not connected with the organization.	Have a well-defined, effective, and practiced security plan.
Type 2	Violence committed by customers, or people connected to the organization.	Have a well-defined, effective, and practiced security plan including a buddy system and crisis intervention and response training.
Type 3	Violence committed by current or former employees.	Have a well-defined, effective, and practiced security plan including a buddy system and crisis intervention and response training. Be aware of warning signs that the employee is in crisis.
Type 4	Violence committed by someone connected to an employee.	Have a well-defined, effective, and practiced security plan including a buddy system and crisis intervention and response training. Be aware of warning signs that the employee is in crisis.

Source: Rugala, EA ed. Workplace Violence, Issues in Response. Washington, DC: U.S. Department of Justice; 2002.

companies in rural America are potential targets. Terrorists may look to large and populous targets as high potential for death and injury; however, small targets in areas not prone to attack may go further toward instilling of terror and panic.[1]

Type 2 violence is perpetrated by a customer of the institution. Customer is used in a very broad sense here and could mean a student, patient, actual customer, anyone receiving some sort of service from an institution or its employee. Those employed by corrections, law enforcement, and health care, especially nurses, are particularly at risk. Violent reactions by customers are unpredictable and may be triggered by excessive waits or dissatisfaction with the level of service. Nurses, physicians, nurse practitioners, and other health-care providers in the mental health, emergency, critical care areas, and crisis intervention areas seem to be most at risk for type 2 violence. A well-thought-out security plan, buddy system, and crisis training including defensive actions are essential to lessening this risk.[1]

Types 3 and 4 violence are either a former employee or domestic partner presenting to the workplace with intent to kill one or many employees. Of all the types of violence mentioned here, it may be the most preventable by paying attention to a few warning signs. Again, strong security plans and protocols are essential to mitigating the potentially disastrous outcome of these events.[1]

Planning for Workplace Violence

Dealing with workplace violence takes the involvement of management, the employees, and the broader community. Violence of this nature affects the whole community through loss of productivity, potential loss of wages, and loss of services in addition to the intangible negative effects of violence on the community as a whole. Although it is the legal and ethical responsibility of management to provide a safe work environment, the cooperation of the whole community is necessary for the prevention of and the response to workplace violence. Planning, therefore, must include management, employees and unions, local law enforcement, and those from mental health and social services.[1,4]

WHY IS IT IMPORTANT To Participate?

Planning must include management, employees and unions, and local law enforcement and those from mental health and social services. Unless all aspects of the work environment are active participants and cooperate to form a plan that meets the needs of everyone involved, it will not be effective.

Employers should develop a clear fair security plan that fosters trust with their employees. The plan should include appropriate discipline measures that should be administered fairly. Once the plan is in place, all current employees should be made aware of it and be part of the orientation of new employees. Regular training sessions should be part of a yearly cycle of employee and management training. The work environment must be conducive to fair treatment of both the victim and the accused. Victims of domestic abuse, when the actions or the results of the actions, follow the victim to work, should not be treated as if they are the cause of the problem. They should be made to feel safe in the work environment. Those accused of perpetrating violence or threats also should be treated fairly. Neither the accused nor the victim should feel that they are improperly treated. To do so continues the violence.[1,4,5]

Planning is difficult. It should not include what has become the current definition of "zero tolerance." Zero tolerance was intended to imply that all threats were to be addressed; it was never intended to mean that all threats were to be treated the same. It may be easy to develop a plan in which any threat be it an off-the-cuff remark in a moment of frustration or one that is significant and specific are dealt with by removing the offending person but it does not make sense from either a fiscal perspective—training new employees is expensive—or in the creation of a fair and comfortable work environment. H. L. Mencken's aphorism: "For every problem, there is a solution which is simple, neat, and wrong." Avoid a one-size-fits-all policy on preventing or reacting to violence.[1]

WHY IS IT IMPORTANT To Address All Threats Appropriately?

Zero tolerance was intended to imply that all threats were to be addressed; it was never intended to mean that all threats were to be treated the same. Ibuprofen is not the same as heroin or crack cocaine. A small pocket knife is not the same as a loaded hand gun and a stolen kiss by a child in kindergarten is not the raping of a 14-year-old adolescent. All threats must be addressed and each should be evaluated based on the level of threat and the intent.

Management should develop the security plan, put it in writing, and distribute it to all management and staff. It should clearly specify that workplace violence does not just mean physical violence but includes threats, bullying, and intimidation. The security plan should encompass prevention and response, being proactive not reactive. The plan must have the support of top executives and employees. It should fit the environment; each workplace has its own needs and culture. Some have high levels of stress whereas others may be relaxed. Some will have close relationships and others may foster limited interaction. The plan should be adaptable over time. As it is implemented, evaluate the result. Change should not come from a knee-jerk reaction but from a thorough evaluation of successes and failures. Practice the plan and include top management in the practice. This process of development and implementation is complex; involve professionals from mental health, emergency response, and law enforcement throughout the process.[1,4,5]

Components of the plan should include the following:

- Prevention, an assessment of the physical security of the organization.
- Written procedures for addressing threats or physical violence.
- Designated personnel from both management and staff who are responsible for response and implementation of the plan and training.
- Crisis response procedures.
- Outside resources available to all employees and management.

Application should be consistent and fair. This plan should complement existing drug and alcohol policies.[1,5]

Prevention

Prevention begins with interviewing potential employees. There is no "type" of person who is guaranteed to be violent at work. People with pasts that include significant encounters with the judicial system and are convicted felons may have changed and will make fine employees, whereas a person from a fine local family may decide to commit horrible acts of violence. Nonetheless, past drug use or violence along with a history of multiple job changes or dismissals may be indicative of a problem employee and should be addressed in the interview. Behavior that is defensive or hostile and responses that blame others for problems and conflicts should raise red flags concerning the appropriateness of an employee.[1]

Violence may affect one employee or the workplace as a whole. Identifying and thereby preventing an employee from perpetrating an act of violence is difficult. As with hiring, there is no profile that definitely indicates a problem. Management should avoid falsely accusing an employee of inappropriate behavior when they have not "crossed the line." It would be better to make the employee aware of concerns and offer counseling and support before the concern escalates to a problem. There are some behaviors and circumstances that may indicate concern. Personality conflicts between employees, mishandled terminations or disciplinary measures, drug or alcohol use at work, or an exaggerated response to real or imagined problems may be circumstances that may escalate into violence. Personal issues such as family problems and frustrations at home may also carry to the workplace. Certain behaviors may also be signs that a problem is beginning to escalate. Employees who become increasingly belligerent, begin to make specific threats, become hypersensitive to criticism, exhibit outbursts of anger, have obsession with a coworker or supervisor, have a noticeable change in behavior, or have suicidal or homicidal ideation should raise red flags. Suicidal ideation is a concern beyond the victim's plans to do harm to themselves because they may intend to harm themselves by being killed during an act of violence or by killing themselves after they have killed others around them.[1]

Although it is impossible and inappropriate to assign blame for triggering an act of violence, there are circumstances that may be seen as instigating violence in the workplace. Understaffing that leads to compulsory overtime and subsequent stress, poor management styles involving discipline and direction, labor disputes, downsizing, or inadequate and poorly trained security staff may lead to employee dissatisfaction and instigate an act of violence.[1]

Physical Security

A survey of the security needs of the institution is essential. Are the entrances visible and well lit? Is the layout of the building such that there are easy exit routes for evacuations? Are there small areas where employees may become trapped? Are there employees with special needs who will need to be helped during an evacuation of the building? Is there an adequate system to notify employees that they must leave the building? Have arrangements been made for all of the employees to gather in specific areas until all have been accounted for, or if there is not a set list of employees present at regular times, is there a mechanism in place to ensure all employees are out of the building? Is the security staff well qualified and trained and do they regularly interact with local law enforcement to familiarize them with the security needs of the organization? After the physical needs are evaluated and a plan for evacuation established it is important to make any changes needed to the physical structure and to practice the evacuation plan regularly.[1,5]

Write It Down

After the plan is established for prevention and response, write it down, practice it, evaluate it and redesign it as needed. Assign specific people to important tasks related to threat assessment, evacuation, crisis management, and response. If the organization is large enough, assign back-up personnel to key positions. Establish committees made up of management and staff to evaluate threats and respond fairly. Practice. It is perhaps hardest to maintain competence in a plan that may be implemented rarely.[1,5]

School Violence

School violence may be more difficult to predict and understand than workplace violence. Again there is no profile of a typical student who will threaten or carry out school mass violence. The profile put forth by the media of a "loner" or problem child is not always the case. Nor is the perception that school mass violence is on the rise. It is usually a devastating and horrendous act garnishing large amount of publicity; it is

Evidence for Practice

There is no profile of a typical student who will threaten or carry out school mass violence. There are things to watch out for and consider, but no definitive profile that will always point to someone planning violence. Analyze every threat, and consider each student individually. Above all, have a plan to deal with threats and with violence should it occur.

also very rare. Misconceptions concerning school mass violence are many:

- All school shooters are loners and alike.
- The acts are motivated by revenge.
- The behavior follows some aberrant interest or hobby and access to weapons is the most significant factor.

In fact, none of these things are consistently true.[6]

Predicting school mass violence is not usually possible. Predicting when or if students who have no history of a violent act will kill their classmates and then themselves is impossible. The outcry from such an event usually demands that "something be done," and often results in a knee-jerk response that never addresses the root of the issues. The community demands stricter laws controlling student behavior, stricter gun control measures, and a show of force in the school in the form of metal detectors and security. Any threat, no matter how slight, is taken as seriously as another. A nail file is as serious as a knife and may cause the student to be expelled. The student who brings an aspirin to school for a headache is treated the same as a student with illegal drugs. Laws and actions such as these are easy to enforce but they do not solve the problems or issues that cause mass school violence. They do nothing to prevent an incident of devastating mass school violence.[6]

Planning for School Mass Violence

Schools are different from workplaces in many ways. There is a sense that there is more control within the environment. Parents, teachers, and administration can easily make rules governing behavior because they are dealing with children not adults. The culture is less about productivity and more about exploration. It is an environment of learning. There is more movement of people and things through the school throughout the day. Students do not act with the same controls as adults. At younger ages, they have not learned all of the social norms most adults live by. As student populations grow older, they begin to feel more and more independent and act accordingly. So while adults may easily make rules to control behavior, students may not always follow them. There are varying levels of control but none are complete.[6]

In general, the same actions that assist in controlling mass violence in the workplace apply to the school. A definite plan written down and practiced that includes prevention, a physical survey of the school, assigned roles for administration, faculty, staff, and students to deal with both the threat and incident of violence should be implemented. As discussed, in both the work and school environments, it is important to take all threats seriously. Everyone in both environments has the right to feel safe. In the school environment, it is difficult to learn when you are concerned about your safety. However, just as in the work environment, not all threats are equal and each should be evaluated on its own merits.[5,6]

Prevention

Most schools have little control over who is eligible to be a student. There may be some limitation factors particularly in private school and colleges or universities; however, these are not the same as a person interviewing for employment. A person does not have a "right to work" whereas children in the United States have a right to go to school. Although there may be structures that can be built into the education system of each school to mitigate problems from segments of students, it is not the place of this book to discuss or comment on their merits.

Just as in the workplace, all threats should be taken seriously and evaluated. Both the perpetrator and victim should be treated fairly and appropriately. Involve parents and children to identify the root of violence and teach problem solving both by word and example. Define what is considered a threat or violence and make all students, faculty, and staff aware. Define the process by which each will be evaluated and what the sanctions will be. Make all faculty, students, staff, parents, and administrators aware of the policy and implement it fairly.[1,6]

Physical Survey

An in-depth survey of the physical layout of the school should be undertaken. Although most administrators may say they know their schools well, there are pockets where students can hide or be trapped. A well-thought-out evacuation plan should be developed and practiced. Faculty and staff should be assigned tasks as part of the plan to make sure all students are out and procedures are in place to account for the students after they have left the building. Plans should be in place to deal specifically with mass violence. It may not be best to have all students rush into the hall; the physical placement and layout may allow some students to leave through first floor windows. Doors may be barred to prevent entry by perpetrators, though this may create problems in a hostage situation.[1,5,6]

In the end, there is not a single plan that will satisfy all situations. Local law enforcement and emergency medical services should be involved in exploring appropriate options. They should be familiar with the physical structure of the building and what steps school personnel will take in the event of violence. They should know if the school attempts to evacuate or lock down and where those who do escape will gather. Whereas it is appropriate to make all employees in a workplace aware of plans to deal with violence, it may or may not be appropriate to make students aware of the specifics of the school's plan. Depending on the specifics, a student who is planning mass violence may be able to use them against others. There is no right or wrong answer nor is there a right or wrong plan, there are only better and best. Any plan is better than no plan; a well-thought-out plan is best.[1,5,6]

Threat Assessment

Threat assessment is the process by which threats are judged for their level or severity. Not all threats are the same. Some threats may be made off the cuff in a moment of frustration during a casual conversation whereas others are thought out, specific, with intent to follow through. Deciding which is difficult; there are significant gray areas. Responding to an act of violence is easier than responding to a threat. Responding to the threat is always preferable to dealing with mass violence.[1]

In either the workplace or school, there should be trained, designated personnel who will evaluate each reported threat. Training should include the following:

- Risk management.
- Crisis management.
- Conflict resolution.
- Understanding of interpersonal relationships.

This may be one school administrator or management member or it may be a team of individuals from multiple levels within the structure of the organization. Personnel involved with security, human resources, legal, health care, and mental health should be involved. Their task may be to interview those involved with the incident, examine past problems and circumstances surrounding the incident, or to refer the case to outside authorities. Theirs is the difficult task of deciding what should be done.[1,6]

Threats then may be classified in four ways: indirect, direct, veiled, and conditional[1,6] **(see Table 7–2).**

- A direct threat indicates a specific act that is planned against a specific institution or person. For instance: "I am going to place a bomb in the cafeteria at lunch. That will teach them a lesson."
- An indirect threat is much less specific. There is vagueness about who, when, and how. For instance: "I could kill everyone here if I wanted to."
- A veiled threat implies violence but does not specifically threaten violence. "We all would be better off without

TABLE 7–2   Types of Threats

TYPE OF THREAT	DEFINITION
Indirect	An indirect threat is much less specific. There is vagueness about whom, when, and how. For instance; "I could kill everyone here if I wanted to."
Direct	A direct threat indicates a specific act that is planned against a specific institution or person. For instance; "I am going to place a bomb in the cafeteria at lunch. That will teach them a lesson."
Veiled	A veiled threat implies violence but does not specifically threaten violence. "We all would be better off without you around."
Conditional	A conditional threat states that a violent act will occur if some demand is not met. "If you don't leave and never come back to school/work, I will kill you."

O'Toole ME. The School Shooter: A Threat Assessment Perspective. Washington, DC: U.S Department of Justice/Federal Bureau of Investigation; 1999.

you around." With both indirect and veiled threats it is suggested that violent acts may occur without saying they will occur.

• A conditional threat states that a violent act will occur if some demand is not met. "If you don't leave and never come back to school/work, I will kill you."

Emotional content and specific precipitating events may seem as if they make threats more likely but this may not be true. What does seem to be true is that the more specific and plausible the details are within the threat, the more likely the threat will be carried out. The details may include the identity of the victim, when and where the threat will be carried out, and how it will be done. Such detail may indicate significant forethought and planning. However, the threat must be plausible. If the details are such that it would be impossible to carry it out, it would seem unlikely that the threat is serious[1,6] (see Table 7–3).

Through analysis, a level of risk may be assigned to a threat. Threats may be seen as low, medium, and high risk. A low-level risk would pose a minimal risk to the victim or victims. The details are vague and indirect or it may be implausible, lacking

TABLE 7–3	Level of Threats	
LEVEL OF THREAT	**DEFINITION**	**ACTION**
Low	A low-level risk would pose a minimal risk to the victim or victims. The details are vague and indirect or it may be implausible, lacking realism. It is unlikely that the threat will be carried out.	Counseling of employee or student and observation.
Medium	A medium-level threat appears to be a threat that could be carried out. It is more direct and specific. There may appear to be more planning and fore-thought with some indication of timing. There may be references to a place and a weapon with a more specific reason or motivation, though all of this will lack the specificity of a high-level threat.	The most difficult to evaluate and act on. The threat should still be taken seriously and counseling of the student or employee and all involved should be the minimum response. Anger management and problem-solving training should be included. Law enforcement may need to be involved.
High	A high-level threat will be very specific. It will be direct, concrete, and plausible. It will specify weapon, place, time, and victim or victims. When to bring in law enforcement is difficult.	Threat should be taken very seriously and considered likely to be carried out. Law enforcement should be involved.

realism. It is unlikely that the threat will be carried out. A medium-level threat appears to be a threat that could be carried out. It is more direct and specific. There may appear to be more planning and fore thought with some indication of timing. There may be references to a place and a weapon with a more specific reason or motivation, though all of this will lack the specificity of a high-level threat. A high-level threat will be very specific. It will be direct, concrete, and plausible. It will specify weapon, place, time, and victim or victims. When to bring in law enforcement is difficult. Certainly, a high-level threat should be taken seriously and should involve law enforcement whereas low-level threats should be examined with steps taken to ensure that the threat is unlikely. Medium-level threats are more of a problem. Again, steps should be taken to minimize the potential of violence and ensure the safety of those involved. The involvement of law enforcement should be strongly considered but it may be difficult to judge the seriousness of the person's intention. In the workplace where you are dealing with adults, involvement of law enforcement may seem appropriate and obvious; when dealing with the emotions and lack of maturity in children, it is not so obvious. A medium-level threat may be just emotional angst or it may be precipitated by the one act that pushes a child to carry out mass violence. Choosing wrongly may either needlessly cause a child to be accused of a crime or allow significant loss of life.[1,6]

Evaluation

The FBI recommends a four-pronged approach specifically for school violence. Adapted to the workplace, it may be able to provide a basis for understanding violence in either the workplace or school and a way to begin to analyze threats in either environment. It includes personality of the student, family dynamics, work or school dynamics, and social dynamics. It should be emphasized again that no one personality trait, family, school, or social dynamic should be considered in isolation will point to a potentially violent person. The whole must be considered when evaluating a situation.[1,6]

Behavior Traits

Following is a partial list of behaviors which should be considered when evaluating a threat:

- **Low Tolerance for Frustration**
  - Although all students and employees feel frustrated at times, those who easily feel they have been wronged by others particularly when the complaints are vague.
- **Poor Coping Skills**
  - Employees and students who seem unable to cope with normal frustrations, failures, wrongs, and humiliations within the school or workplace environment.
- **Lack of Resiliency**
  - Students or employees who are unable to put failures, problems, and humiliations behind them even after a period of time has elapsed.
- **Injustice Collector**
  - Those who collect wrongs, either perceived or real and never resolve the issues; those who hold grudges.
- **Narcissism and Alienation**
  - Employees or students who are self-centered to the extent that they lack insight into others. They feel that they are different from others and embrace the role of victim. They are loners and have a sense of separateness from those around them.
- **Dehumanization and Lack of Empathy**
  - Employees or students who feel that those around them, particularly those who may have wronged them, are non-humans and not worthy of consideration. They do not empathize with other's needs or emotions. As nonhumans, it is okay to harm them.
- **Exaggerated Sense of Entitlement and Superiority**
  - Employees or students who feel that they are significantly better than those around them in every way. They have a sense that they deserve special consideration in all circumstances and feel wronged when they do not receive it.
- **Externalizes Blame**
  - People who believe they are never wrong. If there is a failure, it is the result of actions by someone else. They seem impervious to rational arguments.

- **Intolerance and Inappropriate Humor**
  - Students or employees are intolerant of those different from them. They may use inappropriate slogans or phrases or tell jokes that imply violence against others around them.
- **Lack of Trust, Rigid and Opinionated**
  - Students or employees who are absolutely fixated on their belief structure; no amount of rational discussion will convince them that they are wrong. They feel that there are no trustworthy people or institutions around them. When something happens, they must take care of it themselves. They are the only ones who can right a wrong.

Besides these behaviors, people may be depressed, have anger management issues, have violent role models or idolize violence. Their actions and verbalizations may mask low self-esteem and they may have an exaggerated need for attention. They may exhibit a significant change in behavior and begin to alienate friends or coworkers. Their performance in school or at work may begin to deteriorate.[1,6]

Family Dynamics

The second prong in the evaluation process is an examination of family dynamics. In the case of a student, the family dynamics provide insight into controls, concerns, or problems the child has grown up with. The family may be in turmoil; there may have been a significant change in the family dynamic or the environment may be violent. Parents may have few if any controls over the child and accept violent or pathological behavior. There may be a casualness concerning weapons.[6]

The employee or student may be going through very difficult problems at home. They may be being abused by their significant other or are the ones perpetrating the abuse. Violence may follow them to work or they may begin to take out their frustrations from home at work.

Work or School Environment

The environment the student or employee works in must be considered when evaluating a threat or violence. It may be difficult because neither school administrators and faculty or management wish to see contributing factors for which they are responsible. An environment that tolerates disrespect of authority and disrespect of fellow students or employees by allowing bullying, pecking orders, and a lack of fairness in the application of the rules diminishes learning and productivity and provides a basis for violence and an acceptance of threats.[1,6]

Social Dynamics

The peer groups the student or employee is a part of or the lack of social contact may affect the potential for threats to become violent. If there is a common fascination with violence or drug and alcohol use within the group and no one from the outside to correct the acceptance of this type of behavior, the person may be more inclined to turn a threat into violence. An incident in another school or workplace may cause the person or group to act on a threat, acting as a copycat.[1,6]

As stated, no single item points to a person who is definitely going to commit an act of violence. Each threat must be taken and evaluated upon its merits. No one answer or course of action is appropriate. It may be appropriate to expel or suspend the student or fire the employee; or it may be more appropriate to provide counseling and remedial training. In the case of the student, involve the family and possibly peers in both the evaluation and resolution. If the work or school environment is partially at fault, take corrective actions to improve the environment. Prevention of violence is always preferable to response.[1,6]

Action

There is no one way to respond to mass violence, but there are a few general thoughts and two overriding attitudes. First, always be aware of your surroundings. As described in Chapter 4, being aware of what is right and wrong around you may save your life. Do not get caught unaware and unable to respond. If the day does not feel right, make yourself hyperaware and have a plan of action. If nothing happens, laugh and relax, if something does, you will stand a better chance of surviving.

WHY IS IT IMPORTANT | To Act With Intensity?

Whatever you do, do it with the intensity of the sun. We do not approach many things in life with such intensity. We say we give something 100% or say we did something as if our life depended on it, but we rarely do. In situations where we are in fact fighting for our lives we must act accordingly. Speak with absolute sincerity, fight without any rules, and do not stop until the threat is either gone or long past down, run until you collapse, and if you hide, in your mind you must be infinitely small. Life is not like the movies; the perpetrators do not always fall down when you hit them and the good guys do not always show up at the last second. Try to survive with everything you have.

Second, if something does happen, do whatever you decide to do with an intensity like you have never experienced before. Life is not like the movies, you should not hit an assailant one time and expect him to fall to the ground while you walk away. Whatever you do, do with the intensity of the sun. Be absolutely relentless in carrying out your actions. This is difficult. We often say we give 100%, but it is unlikely unless you have been in a life-threatening situation, such as combat, that you have truly given 100%. If you are fighting for your life, put all the preconceived notions you may have seen in the movies aside and act until you are free or dead.

As to how you should act, there is no right or wrong and every set of circumstances is different. You may not be physically able to leave or you may feel a sense of responsibility to students or others around you. You may be carrying a firearm, if the environment you are in allows you to and you are legally able to, so you may feel you can resolve the situation, you may not. You may have other training or responsibilities that compel certain actions. Life is fluid with an infinite number of possible choices and actions.

In general, if you can get out, you should get out. Not being in the presence of danger is the best way to avoid danger. Do not just run in a panic; be aware of where you are running and where you need to go. Be aware of who is around you, they may be able to help you or you them, but as you run, run with the intensity of the sun. If you cannot escape, the next safest choice is to hide. Here too, if you hide, be aware of what is going on around you, do not panic or freeze, but decide how and where to hide. Barricade yourself and possibly others in an area where you can absolutely control access. Remember, that although the tool of most mass violence is a gun, there are other weapons that the assailant may employ, such as fire. If you hide, hide with the intensity of the sun. The most dangerous choice is to fight, either verbally or physically. This increases your chances of being hurt significantly, but you may not have a choice. If the perpetrator engages those around him or her in conversation, talk to them and remember, there are no rules. This is not like the movies where you are going to make some promise only if you can carry it out. Be absolutely sincere and say whatever you need to say to convince them to give themselves up. Remember, you are fighting using your words as weapons; they may be silent, soft, or loud, understand and respond to the perpetrator. If you find yourself having to physically fight the perpetrator, again there are no rules. Do not panic, but act in any and every way possible to overcome the assailant. Attack sensitive parts of the body: the eyes, the groin, knees, and tops of the feet. Do not strike once and expect the assailant to stop. If you start fighting, continue until the assailant is dead or incapacitated and can be restrained. Fight only as a last resort, but if you do, fight with the intensity of the sun.

Summary

In the end, do not panic, if local law enforcement is involved with planning, use them to help map out the type of response the employees or students should take. Specifically how individuals should respond must be a part of the plan and each part should work in concert to protect everyone in the building. Do not be inflexible, practice the plan, and see where it works, where it fails, and how it should be changed. If an event should occur, adapt the plan as necessary and survive. Above all, don't panic.

1. Rugala EA, ed. Workplace Violence, Issues in Response. Washington, DC: U.S. Department of Justice; 2002.
2. Hogan DE, Burnstein JL, eds. *Disaster Medicine*. 2002, Philadelphia, PA: Lippincott Williams & Wilkins; 2002:432.
3. Anderson C, Parish M. Report of workplace violence by Hispanic nurses. *Journal of Transcultural Nursing*. 2003;14(3):237–243.
4. Levin PF, Hewitt JB, Misner ST. Insights of nurses about assault in hospital-based emergency departments.[see comment]. *Image—Journal of Nursing Scholarship*. 1998;30(3):249–254.
5. Wilkinson CW. Violence prevention at work. A business perspective. *American Journal of Preventive Medicine*. 2001;20(2):155–160.
6. O'Toole ME. The School Shooter: A Threat Assessment Perspective. Washington, DC: U.S Department of Justice/ Federal Bureau of Investigation; 1999.

Biological Agents 8

Introduction

Nursing and other health-care providers must become well informed concerning the use of biological agents as terrorist agents or because of accidental releases; either may have devastating effects on local, national, or worldwide populations. Student nurses and student advanced practice nurses (APN) should become familiar with the presentation of these rarely seen diseases, their treatment, and the protective equipment required by each agent within their respective programs of study. Practicing nurses and APNs need to be vigilant concerning outbreaks. Many agents spread quickly and can be devastating. Treatment protocols should be implemented quickly if an outbreak is suspected to minimize the spread of the disease and its long-term effects. Medical and nursing care provided by nurses, APNs, and other health-care providers is essential to establish positive outcomes. This includes knowing when to isolate your patient, providing good respiratory care, antibiotic therapy, minimizing stress on septic patients, fluid and electrolyte monitoring and treatment, and knowing how to protect contacts and those providing care.

Administrators need to provide the means to accomplish these goals. Proper protective equipment and facilities are essential. Hospital staff should receive regular continuing education to maintain competencies concerning the recognition and treatment of these rare diseases. This may be difficult with many competing needs both educationally and financially but remains important. Lastly, administration should provide opportunities for nursing and medical staff to practice these skills and knowledge through drills, table top exercises, and case studies.

Biological agents are defined as any bacteria, virus, or toxin from bacteria that are used to cause illness or death either purposely as from terrorists or from an accidental release. History documents the use of biological agents used to cause illness, death, and panic dating as early as the 14th century when the Tartars catapulted victims of the plague into the city Kaffa, fleas then spread the plague throughout Europe causing the Black Death. The Russians used the same tactics against the Swedes during the Russian-Swedish war of 1700–1725. The English gave blankets contaminated with small pox to Native Americans during the French and Indian war. The Japanese used plague-infested fleas against the Chinese during the 1930s and 1940s. Although the Biological Weapons Convention treaty was signed by the United States, Soviet Union, and one hundred other nations in 1972, clandestine efforts to cultivate and weaponize biological agents continued **(see Fig. 8–1).**

Biological agents with terrorist potential may be naturally endemic to an area and cause limited outbreaks. Others are tightly controlled and may only cause an incident from an intentional release. *Yersinia pestis*, the plague, occurs naturally in many parts of the world and botulism has caused outbreaks related to improperly canned food. Conversely, small pox was eradicated in 1980. Any outbreak of small pox today could not be a natural occurrence; it would have to be related to an accidental or unintentional release from one of the two remaining storage sites in either the United States or the former Soviet Union.

WHY IS IT IMPORTANT **To Be Knowledgeable About Biological Agents?**

Intentional release of biological agents could cause significant morbidity and mortality in addition to widespread panic and social disruption. The diseases they cause are rare and may be difficult to recognize making appropriate treatment and containment difficult and resulting in spread beyond the initial outbreak.

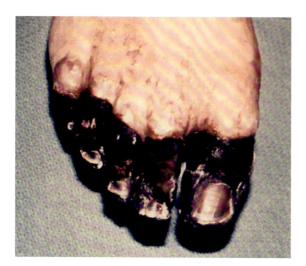

FIGURE 8–1. This patient presented with symptoms of plague that included gangrene of the right foot causing necrosis of the toes. In this case, the presence of systemically disseminated plague bacteria *Y. pestis*, that is septicemia, predisposed this patient to abnormal coagulation within the blood vessels of his toes. *Photo courtesy of the Public Health Images Library, CDC.*

As agents of terror, biological agents are extremely effective. They are invisible to the naked eye and, depending on the agent, may spread as easily as through a cough. These agents can cause widespread panic and social disruption based on both the illness and the panic it causes. Though perhaps uniquely qualified to cause panic and disruption, there are problems that make development and dissemination of biological agents difficult. A sufficient quantity of the agent would need to be produced in an effective weaponized form. The agent would need to be dispersed over a large, well-populated area in a manner that effectively inoculates the intended victims. The development, storage, and dissemination all must be done undetected without accidental, premature exposure or exposure of the terrorist. In a world ever more prone to suicide attacks, this last point may be less of a concern to terrorists.[1–4]

There are several agents that the Centers for Disease Control and Prevention (CDC) has designated as high risk for use as a terrorist weapon **(see Table 8–1).** The designation is based on several factors: ease of production, ease of dissemination, and the ability to cause morbidity and mortality, and panic. The agents are anthrax, small pox, plague, botulism, tularemia, and viral hemorrhagic fever **(Table 8–1).** Of these, anthrax, plague, and tularemia are bacterial. Small pox and viral hemorrhagic fever are caused by viruses and, lastly, botulism is caused by a toxin produced by bacteria. All of these are reportable to local public health and the CDC. These agents, their signs and symptoms, and their treatments will each be discussed in this chapter.

Anthrax

Bacillus anthracis is the bacterium that causes the disease anthrax. Anthrax derives its name from the Greek *anthrakis* meaning coal because of the black, coal-like lesions caused by cutaneous anthrax. Anthrax has been known since ancient times, both the Greeks and Egyptians wrote about it. In the Middle Ages it was known as the "Black Bane." A vaccine was developed in 1880, and became the first disease, after small pox, to have an effective vaccine.[4]

ALERT!

The most recent use of a biological agent as a terrorist act was inhalation anthrax, causing 23 victims and five deaths. The vector for spreading the spores was the United States Postal Service. 33,000 people required prophylactic antibiotic treatment. Many of these agents, including anthrax, can be difficult to weaponize and spread effectively; however, each can be devastating once processed and spread. Postal workers were exposed to anthrax simply from processing the mail. The buildings involved in the attacks required the work of hundreds of contractors over a 6-month period at a cost of 3 billion dollars to the post office and 24 million dollars to the United States government to clean up and reopen some of the buildings.

TABLE 8–1 Biological Agents With Terrorist Potential Listed by the Center for Disease Control and Prevention

	AGENT	HUMAN-TO-HUMAN INFECTION	VACCINE	TREATMENT	INCUBATION PERIOD
BACTERIA					
Anthrax	*Bacillus anthracis*	No	Limited	Antibiotic therapy	Inhaled—hours to 60 days Cutaneous—1 to 12 days
Tularemia	*Francisella tularensis*	No, strict laboratory precautions	Limited	Antibiotic therapy	3 to 6 days
Plague	*Yersinia pestis*	Yes	No	Antibiotic therapy	Bubonic—2 to 6 days Pneumonic—1 to 3 days
VIRUS					
Small pox	Small pox virus	Yes	Limited	Supportive therapy	7 to 17 days
Viral hemorrhagic fever	Filoviridae, Arenaviridae, Bunyaviridae, and Flaviviridae	Yes	No	Supportive therapy	5 to 17 days
TOXINS					
Botulism	*Clostridium botulinum*	No	No	Trivalent antitoxin A, B, E. Antitoxin A, B, C, D, E, F, G available through the military	Progressive

Anthrax occurs naturally when herbivores such as cattle and sheep consume grasses grown on soil contaminated with anthrax bacteria. It is a naturally occurring bacterium in soil; animals may sicken and die after eating the grass. Human contact with contaminated animal products also may become infected. The disease has been reported in more than 80 countries. Human-to-human infection has not been reported. Cutaneous anthrax is the most common reported form whereas inhalation anthrax is quite rare; inhaled anthrax would likely be the route chosen by terrorists[1,2,4–8] **(see Fig. 8–2).**

During World War II, it was reported that the Japanese infected prisoners of war and Chinese civilians with anthrax. Both the United States and Soviet Union produced weapon-grade stockpiles of anthrax throughout the cold war period. Iraq also was reported to have stockpiled anthrax. The Japanese cult Aum Shinrikyo attempted to use anthrax in a terrorist attack in 1993. In 2001, anthrax spores

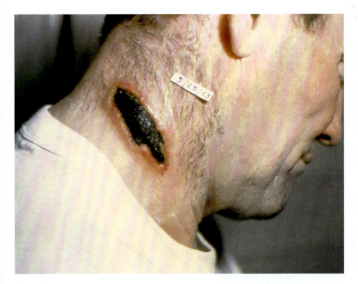

FIGURE 8–2. Cutaneous anthrax lesion on the neck of a victim. Note the black necrotic center from which anthrax takes its name. *Photo courtesy of the Public Health Images Library, CDC.*

were mailed in threatening letters to Tom Browkaw and U.S. Senators Daschle and Leahy. As a result of this incident, 23 victims contracted the disease and five died. The anthrax bacilli cannot survive outside of its host because it requires an environment rich in amino acids and glucose; when these are exhausted or when exposed to air, it forms spores. These spores are extremely hardy, difficult to destroy, and may survive for decades in a typical environment.[1,3,4]

Signs and Symptoms

Anthrax affects animals primarily as gastrointestinal anthrax. In humans, there are three forms depending on how the spores enter the body. They are cutaneous, inhaled, and gastrointestinal.[1,2,6,8]

- **Cutaneous anthrax:** Cutaneous anthrax accounts for 95% of reported cases. The spores infect the victim by entering through breaks in the skin. A painless lesion develops with black eschar at the center. The lesion usually remains localized, though if untreated systemic infection may develop. Incubation periods range from 1 to 12 days. The lesion begins as a painless, pruritic macular or papular lesion, much like an insect bite. By day two the lesion has swollen, vesiculates, and ruptures to form depressed ulcer. Smaller lesions may form around the primary lesion. The clear serosanguineous fluid in these lesions contains large quantities of the bacilli. The area surrounding the lesion will be swollen. The black eschar forms over the depression, dries, and falls off in 1 to 2 weeks. Lesions affecting the head and neck may have significant swelling.[1,2,4,6,8,9]
- **Inhaled anthrax:** Inhaled anthrax presents as a biphasic disease. The initial phase begins with flu-like symptoms

Evidence for Practice

Anthrax is not contagious from person to person. Standard body fluid precautions in general should be used when treating victims of anthrax.

including: fever, chills, headache, malaise, muscle aches, weakness, nonproductive cough, and possibly, chest or abdominal discomfort. A short latent period, in which the victim may feel somewhat better, follows and lasts hours to days. The second phase is significantly worse, often leading to death. There is a sudden onset of high fever, diaphoresis, dyspnea, cyanosis, and shock; death may occur in 24 to 36 hours. About 50% of inhaled anthrax cases develop anthrax meningitis. It is indistinguishable from other forms of meningitis and is almost always fatal. The incubation period for inhaled anthrax from exposure to onset of symptoms may be as short as a few hours or as long as 60 days.[1,2,4,6,8]

- **Gastrointestinal anthrax:** Gastrointestinal anthrax is the rarest of the three forms. It can further be broken down into abdominal anthrax and oropharyngeal anthrax. Both occur from eating contaminated meat; the location of the disease is dependent on where the spores germinate. Gastrointestinal anthrax is characterized by fever, malaise, nausea, vomiting, and anorexia, again, much like the flu. This progresses to severe bloody diarrhea, acute abdominal distress, and sepsis. Lesions forming in the gastrointestinal tract will form ulcers and may produce hematemesis. Massive ascites may occur, as will hemorrhagic mesenteric lymphangitis. Blood loss, and fluid and electrolyte imbalances will occur. Death from perforated bowel and toxemia occurs in 2 to 5 days. Mortality is 50%. Oropharyngeal anthrax presents with fever, malaise, and dysphagia. Lesions form in the oral cavity and oropharynx. Swelling may be significant and may compromise the victims' airway. **See Table 8–2** for the various forms of anthrax, their signs and symptoms, and recommended treatment.[1,2,4,6,8]

Evidence for Practice

Diagnosis of anthrax may be difficult because it presents in a manner similar to many respiratory diseases. One significant finding is a widened mediastinum found on chest x-ray. This is key to the diagnosis of inhalation anthrax.

TABLE 8–2 Types of Anthrax With Signs, Symptoms, and Treatment

TYPE	SIGNS AND SYMPTOMS	TREATMENT
Cutaneous anthrax	Begins as a painless pruritic macular or papular lesion. Day two the lesion has swollen, vesiculates and ruptures to form depressed ulcer, black eschar forms over the depression, dries, and falls off in 1 to 2 weeks.	Ciprofloxacin 500 mg every 12 hours for adults or doxycycline 100 mg every 12 hours. Duration is 60 days. Children should receive ciprofloxacin 10–15 mg/kg every 12 hours or doxycycline. Doxycycline should be dosed as follows: >8 yr and >45 kg 100 mg every 12 hours; >8 yr and ≤45 kg 2.2 mg/kg every 12 hours; ≤8 yr 2.2 mg/kg every 12 hours. No change for pregnancy.
Inhaled anthrax	**Phase 1:** fever, chills, headache, malaise, muscle aches, weakness, nonproductive cough, and possibly, chest or abdominal discomfort. **Phase 2:** sudden onset of high fever, diaphoresis, dyspnea, cyanosis, and shock; death may occur in 24–36 hours.	Ciprofloxacin 400 mg every 12 hours for adults or doxycycline 100 mg every 12 hours. Duration is 60 days. Children should receive ciprofloxacin 10–15 mg/kg every 12 hours or doxycycline. Doxycycline should be dosed as follows: >8 yr and >45 kg 100 mg every 12 hours; >8 yr and ≤45 kg 2.2 mg/kg every 12 hours; ≤8 yr 2.2 mg/kg every 12 hours. No change for pregnancy. Treatment should include two additional antibiotics such as chloramphenicol. Fever control, fluid and electrolyte balance, and pain control.

Continued

TABLE 8–2   Types of Anthrax With Signs, Symptoms, and Treatment—cont'd

TYPE	SIGNS AND SYMPTOMS	TREATMENT
Gastrointestinal anthrax	Fever, malaise, nausea, vomiting, anorexia, severe bloody diarrhea, acute abdominal distress, and sepsis.	Ciprofloxacin 400 mg every 12 hours for adults or doxycycline 100 mg every 12 hours. Duration is 60 days.
		Children should receive ciprofloxacin 10–15 mg/kg every 12 hours or doxycycline. Doxycycline should be dosed as follows: >8 yr and >45 kg 100 mg every 12 hours; >8 yr and ≤45 kg 2.2 mg/kg every 12 hours; ≤8 yr 2.2 mg/kg every 12 hours.
		No change for pregnancy.
		Treatment should include two additional antibiotics such as chloramphenicol.
		Fever control, fluid and electrolyte balance, and pain control.

All suspected cases of anthrax must be reported to local and state health departments. The diagnosis must be confirmed by the CDC. Laboratory specimens should be handled according to BSL2 standards.

Treatment

Standard aerobic blood cultures are the most useful diagnostic test for most hospital laboratories. Culture growth should begin in about 6 to 24 hours. Colony morphology and biochemical testing should provide a preliminary diagnosis in 12 to 24 hours. Gram stain of vesicular fluid from cutaneous anthrax also could confirm the diagnosis. This fluid should be cultured. Sputum cultures are not effective. Peripheral blood smears should show gram-positive bacilli with systemic anthrax. Immune histochemical examination of fluid with direct fluorescence assay staining for polysaccharide cell wall and capsule also would confirm diagnosis. Polymerase chain reaction (PCR) would confirm the diagnosis but may not be available at all laboratories.[1,2,4,6,8]

Chest x-rays can be very helpful in the diagnosis of inhaled anthrax. The classic appearance of a widened mediastinum in a patient previously healthy and now symptomatic is very indicative of inhalation anthrax. There also may be hemorrhagic pleural effusions, air bronchograms, or consolidations. Chest x-rays or computed tomography (CT) examinations are key in the diagnosis of inhaled anthrax[1,2,4,6,8] (see Fig. 8–3).

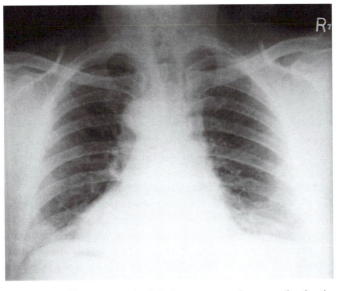

FIGURE 8–3. This posteroanterior (PA) chest x-ray was taken 4 months after the onset of anthrax in a 46-year-old male. This patient had worked for 2 years as a card tender in a goat hair processing mill. X-rays revealed bilateral pulmonary effusion and a widened mediastinum, which are hallmarks of the disease process. *Photo courtesy of the Public Health Images Library, CDC.*

Treatment should always be confirmed with the CDC. Current guidelines for inhaled or systemic anthrax include ciprofloxacin 400 mg every 12 hours for adults. Therapy should begin as an IV infusion but may be switched to oral ciprofloxacin 500 mg when appropriate. Doxycycline 100 mg every 12 hours may be substituted for ciprofloxacin. One or two other antimicrobials should also be used in conjunction with either ciprofloxacin or doxycycline. Treatment should continue for 60 days.

Children should receive ciprofloxacin 10–15 mg/kg every 12 hours or doxycycline. Doxycycline should be dosed as follows: >8 yr and >45 kg 100 mg every 12 hours, >8 yr and <45 kg 2.2 mg/kg every 12 hours, <8 yr 2.2 mg/kg every 12 hours. Again one or two antimicrobials should be added to the course of treatment. Therapy should continue for 60 days. Women who are pregnant should receive the same therapy as the risk from anthrax outweighs the risks from the medications. However, doxycycline should be avoided if at all possible. There are no changes for immune-compromised individuals. Cutaneous anthrax should be treated as previously discussed except that therapy begins as an oral medication. Duration is again 60 days.[1,2,4,6,8]

Ciprofloxacin is not usually recommended for children under 16 years of age; doxycycline also holds risks for children. Of the two medications, ciprofloxacin is preferred for children. If susceptibility testing on cultures confirms that amoxicillin may be used, it becomes the preferred treatment for children. It also may be substituted for ciprofloxacin for pregnant women.[1,2,4,6,8]

If meningitis is suspected, doxycycline should not be used. Ciprofloxacin IV and chloramphenicol becomes the treatment of choice. In the event of a mass exposure in which large numbers of victims will need treatment, oral therapy should be instituted and continued. Those who come in contact with victims of anthrax need not to be treated with prophylaxis antibiotic therapy.[1,2,4,6,8]

There is a vaccine available to a limited group of people including military personnel, laboratory workers, veterinarians, hazardous material personnel, and livestock handlers. It is a series of three injections over 4 weeks. Annual booster is recommended.[4]

Plague remains an endemic disease in several parts of the world today though rarely in the United States. It has been reportedly used as a terrorist weapon in ancient times, though it is more likely that the pandemics that followed these terrorist acts were caused by the fleas from infected rats. This is the preferred manner in which the disease is spread. It is also reported that the Japanese experimented with plague-infected fleas released over Chinese cities during World War II and the former Soviet Union had extensive stockpiles of and research on the plague.[1,2,4,8]

Plague is caused by the gram-negative coccobacillus *Yersinia pestis*. Unlike anthrax, *Y. pestis* does not produce spores and person-to-person transmission is possible. Plague epidemics begin when the rodent population on which the fleas normally feed begins to die off and the fleas begin to feed off of humans. When the flea bites, plague bacteria mix with the blood and is regurgitated back into the victim. This, along with excrement from the flea, infects the victim. Each bite can inoculate a victim with up to thousands of bacteria; as few as 1 to 10 organisms are necessary to cause disease. The victim also may contract the disease from handling or eating infected meat.[1,2,4,6,8]

The bacteria infect the lymphatic system, depositing in regional lymph nodes. In approximately 2 to 8 days, the bacteria multiply causing lymphadenitis, which is manifested as the characteristic bubo. The bacteria eventually destroy the lymph node structure causing bacteremia and septicemia. The spleen, liver, lungs, skin, and mucous membranes are affected. The bacteria also produce an endotoxin that contributes to the progression of the disease. Eventually, disseminated intravascular coagulation (DIC), shock, and coma occur. The bubonic form of plague is the most common, accounting for up to 85% of all cases. A secondary pneumonic form develops when the bacteria from the bubonic form infect the lungs[1,2,4,6,8] **(see Fig. 8–4).**

- **Septicemia plague** accounts for approximately 15% of the cases. It is manifested by gram-negative sepsis without development of the bubo.

- **Pneumonic plague** is caused by the inhalation of the bacteria or secondary to primary bubonic plague. It accounts for only 2% of the cases of plague.
- **Plague meningitis** has symptoms similar to other forms of meningitis and is often found in children after ineffective treatment of another form of plague.
- **Pharyngeal plague** is extremely rare and is the result of the inhalation of bacteria or ingestion of meat infected with bacteria. It manifests in a way similar to tonsillitis with cervical lymphadenopathy and a cervical bubo.

Signs and Symptoms

Plague manifests with headache, fever, chills, malaise, and exhaustion. With bubonic form, buboes form down the lymphatic system from the flea bite, most often in the femoral or

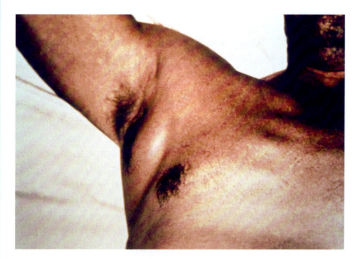

FIGURE 8–4. Plague patient displaying a swollen axillary lymph node. After the incubation period of 2 to 6 days, symptoms of the plague appeared including severe malaise, headache, shaking chills, fever, and pain and swelling, or adenopathy, in the affected regional lymph nodes, also known as buboes. *Photo courtesy of the Public Health Images Library, CDC.*

Evidence for Practice

Plague manifests with headache, fever, chills, malaise, and exhaustion; much like the flu. It then takes the form of bubonic, pneumonic, or septicemic. Plague is endemic to many parts of the world. Large outbreaks in a developed country where it is not endemic should be investigated as a terrorist act.

inguinal areas. They range in size from 1 to 10 cm and are extremely painful. The buboes are not fluctuant but may point, open, and drain spontaneously. Necrosis is rare. If the buboes do not drain, they will require incision and drainage. If septicemia develops it will mimic meningococcemia. Small artery thrombosis will develop in the nose and digits. Appendages will become necrotic; more proximal purpuric lesions will develop. Gangrene is a late finding of the disease progression.[1,2,4,6,8]

Pneumonic plague begins much the same way. No buboes develop; instead, the patient develops a cough hemoptysis, chest pain, dyspnea, stridor, and cyanosis. Death is the result of respiratory failure, bleeding, and circulatory collapse.[1,2,4,6,8]

Patients suspected of plague are infectious to others around them. They should be kept in isolation until 48 hours after antibiotics are instituted. Universal precautions are sufficient for all patients with plague. Those treating patients with pneumonic plague should add disposable surgical masks. Patients being transported also should wear masks[1,2,4,6,8] (see Fig. 8–5).

Treatment

Antibiotic treatment of plague remains streptomycin with gentamicin as first alternative choice. Beyond this, doxycycline, ciprofloxacin, or chloramphenicol may be used. These also are the treatment choices for children. With pregnancy, the first choice is gentamicin, with doxycycline or ciprofloxacin as an alternative. In a mass casualty setting, doxycycline or ciprofloxacin, given orally for adults, children, and pregnant women, is the first choice. Chloramphenicol

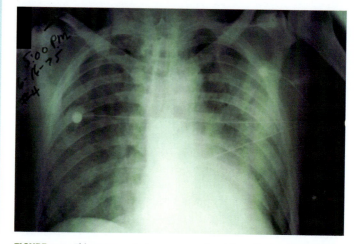

FIGURE 8–5. This anteroposterior x-ray reveals a bilaterally progressive plague infection involving both lung fields. The first signs of plague are fever, headache, weakness, and rapidly developing pneumonia with shortness of breath, chest pain, cough, and sometimes bloody or watery sputum, eventually progressing for 2 to 4 days into respiratory failure and shock. *Photo courtesy of the Public Health Images Library, CDC.*

may be used as an alternative. All antibiotic treatment should ultimately be based on culture sensitivity. Those living in proximity (contact within 2 meters of infected individuals) should receive prophylaxis antibiotics for 7 days and be monitored for fever and cough. Any person developing fever and cough in a mass casualty setting should receive parenteral antibiotics.[1,2,4,6,8]

See Table 8–3 for a listing of types of plague and their signs and symptoms.

The most likely route a terrorist group would use for infecting large groups of people would be through aerosolized distribution of the bacteria. As with other agents, the incubation period and the increased likelihood of travel during this period could create a widespread outbreak as a result. It is also a disease not seen often in most parts of the world and may be misdiagnosed. Plague as a disease instills fear, which easily may cause widespread panic. These reasons make plague a potentially significant weapon of terror.

TABLE 8–3   Manifestations of Plague With Signs and Symptoms

TYPE	SIGNS AND SYMPTOMS
Bubonic plague	Headache, fever, chills, malaise, and exhaustion progressing to disseminated intravascular coagulation (DIC), shock, and coma; buboes form down the lymphatic system from the flea bite 1 to 10 cm and is extremely painful.
Pneumonic plague	Headache, fever, chills, malaise, exhaustion, cough hemoptysis, chest pain, dyspnea, stridor, and cyanosis. Death is the result of respiratory failure, bleeding, and circulatory collapse.
Septicemic plague	Headache, fever, chills, malaise, and exhaustion progressing to gram-negative sepsis without development of the bubo.
Treatment	Streptomycin with gentamicin as first alternative choice. Beyond this, doxycycline, ciprofloxacin, or chloramphenicol may be used.
	Fever control, fluid and electrolyte balance, and pain control.
	Standard Universal Precautions with droplet protection.

Tularemia

Tularemia is endemic to most parts of the world, including the United States. It is a highly virulent disease requiring only a small number of organisms to cause infection. The disease has a very high morbidity imposing significant illness for a significant period of time. Its natural vector is through con- taminated meat or by insect bite. *Francisella tularensis*, the bacteria causing tularemia, is extremely hardy and survives even frigid conditions for years. Aerosolized, it could affect large numbers of victims and contaminate the environment for very long periods of time.[1,2,4,6,8]

Tularemia, *continued*

Evidence for Practice

Tularemia is extremely virulent causing significant morbidity and mortality. Large numbers of victims would be incapacitated for long periods of time. A large outbreak would cause significant social and economic disruption through loss of work, increased health-care needs, and providing care for large numbers of very sick victims for months.

Tularemia presents with nonspecific flu-like illness after a 3- to 6-day incubation period. Fever, chills, myalgias, cough, fatigue, and sore throat is the initial presentation. Patients may experience a pulse rate not in line with a normal rapid pulse consistent with fever. The disease then progresses to ulceroglandular, oculoglandular, tularemic pneumonia, oropharyngeal, or typhoidal tularemia[1,2,4,6,10] **(see Table 8–4).**

Signs and Symptoms

Ulceroglandular tularemia is manifest by ulcerative lesions on the skin or mucous membranes with lymphadenopathy. The lesions range in size from 0.5 to 10 cm. They have a

TABLE 8–4	Manifestations of Tularemia With Signs and Symptoms
TYPE	**SIGNS AND SYMPTOMS**
Prodromal period	Fever, chills, myalgias, cough, fatigue, and sore throat. Patients may experience a pulse rate not in line with a normal rapid pulse consistent with fever.
Ulceroglandular	Ulcerative lesions on the skin or mucous membranes with lymphadenopathy. The lesions range in size from 0.5 to 10 cm.
Oculoglandular	Lesions appear on the eye with purulent conjunctivitis, chemosis, and significant pain.
Tularemic Pneumonia	Worsening cough, dyspnea, chest pain, and hemoptysis.
Oropharyngeal	Pharyngitis, stomatitis, and cervical lymphadenopathy, much like a typical strep pharyngitis.

TABLE 8–4   Manifestations of Tularemia With Signs and Symptoms–cont'd

TYPE	SIGNS AND SYMPTOMS
Typhoidal	Systemic illness without a known source of infection presenting febrile, obtunded, and hypotensive, progresses to shock, multiorgan failure, disseminated intravascular coagulation (DIC), renal failure, meningitis, and death.
Treatment	Streptomycin or gentamicin. Alternative treatment is doxycycline, ciprofloxacin, or chloramphenicol.
	Fever control, fluid and electrolyte balance, and pain control.

granulomatous base with induration. Oculoglandular is similar except that the lesions appear on the eye with purulent conjunctivitis, chemosis, and significant pain. Glandular tularemia has all of the signs and symptoms without lesions. Left untreated, the lymph nodes will drain through the skin. These are the most common presentations of the disease[1,2,6,8,10] (see Fig. 8–6).

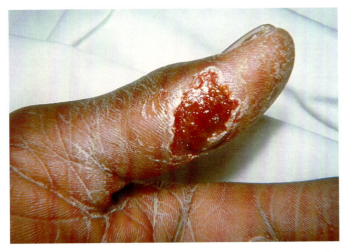

FIGURE 8–6. Thumb with skin ulcer of tularemia. *Photo courtesy of the Public Health Images Library, CDC.*

Oropharyngeal tularemia presents with pharyngitis, stomatitis, and cervical lymphadenopathy, much like a typical strep pharyngitis. Ulcerations may form in the oropharyngeal area. The patient also may complain of abdominal pain, nausea, vomiting, and diarrhea. The usual route of infection for the pathogen is infected meat.[1,2,6,8,10]

Tularemic pneumonia occurs as a result of inhalation of the pathogens. It is speculated that this would be the easiest and most likely form of intentional infection. It occurs naturally in approximately half of all cases of tularemia. The initial symptoms are the same as in other forms with a worsening cough and other respiratory symptoms. Dyspnea, chest pain, and hemoptysis worsen. On chest radiograph, the patient will exhibit bilateral patchy infiltrates, lobar consolidations, and possibly effusions. Hilar lymphadenopathy also may be evident. Untreated, this will worsen to respiratory failure.[1,2,6,8,10]

Typhoidal tularemia is a systemic illness without a known source of infection. Patients are febrile, obtunded, and hypotensive, progressing to shock, multiorgan failure, DIC, renal failure, meningitis, and death. Untreated this has a 60% mortality.[1,2,6,8]

Treatment

Routine laboratory studies including a complete blood count (CBC) and cultures may not be helpful. Because of the high virulence of tularemia, few laboratories may be equipped to handle suspected cases. CBC may only show a mild leukocytosis with lymphocytosis. Chest radiographs are described previously and may not be specific. Latex agglutination and enzyme-linked immunosorbent assays may be helpful when available; however, the antibodies required for this test may take days to weeks to develop.[1,2,6,8,10]

Diagnosis is initially based on clinical suspicion. Presentations of large numbers of previously healthy individuals in a specific geographical area with systemic or respiratory illness, atypical pneumonia with hilar lymphadenopathy should be suspect. If a deliberate infection is suspected, it is reportable to the health department, law enforcement, and the CDC.

First-choice antibiotic treatment is streptomycin or Gentamicin. Alternative treatment is doxycycline, ciprofloxacin, or chloramphenicol. In a mass casualty event, doxycycline 100 mg orally twice a day, ciprofloxacin 500 mg orally twice a day or for children doxycycline 2.2 mg/kg, orally twice a day or ciprofloxacin 15 mg/kg, orally twice a day should be administered for 14 days. Prophylaxis treatment for asymptomatic victims known to be exposed to tularemia is doxycycline or ciprofloxacin as described.[1,2,6,8,10,11]

No human-to-human transmission has been reported so only universal precautions are necessary. Laboratory workers, however, are at risk when handling specimens. Face masks, gowns and gloves should be worn and the specimens should be handled under negative pressure biological cabinets.[1,2,6,8,10]

Tularemia is a virulent bacterial disease with significant morbidity and mortality. It places a significant disease burden on its victims. If released as an aerosol over a well-populated area, it would cause large numbers of victims to become ill for a considerable period of time, causing significant social disruption. As a terrorist weapon, it is not as well known as other agents, but in an intentional release, the potential for widespread panic and disruption remains.

Small Pox

Small pox was eradicated as a disease in 1980. Unfortunately, both the United States and the former Soviet Union retained stockpiles of the virus. Since eradication of the disease, mass vaccinations of the public have stopped. Aside from some possible weak residual immunity in those who received the vaccine years ago, the world population is completely unprepared for an intentional or accidental release of small pox. Stockpiles of small pox vaccine are limited and a significant amount of time would be required to bring facilities online to develop a safe, effective vaccine for mass distribution. This places world populations at even greater risk.[1,2,4,8]

Signs and Symptoms

Exposure to small pox is most often through the respiratory system. The virus then replicates in the local lymph nodes and spreads. A viremia develops throughout the lymph system and seeds the spleen and bone marrow. A secondary viremia seeds the skin and the back of the throat. A prodromal period involving fever, nausea, vomiting, and headache is followed in 2 to 3 days by the characteristic rash. The rash begins on the face followed by the extremities. The rash has a centrifugal appearance unlike varicella (chicken pox), which is more central. The lesions from small pox also progress in unison from macula to vesicle, umbilicated pustula, and finally scab. Patients with chicken pox will have lesions of all forms at the same time. Chicken pox ceases to be infectious after the scabs are formed whereas small pox scabs remain infectious.[1,2,4,8]

Flat-type small pox is a very rare form of the disease. It is characterized by a rapid progression to sepsis. The rash develops slowly, becomes confluent, and remains flat. The lesions never form the crusty lesions normally seen in small pox. Skin may slough off from the areas of the body affected by the rash. Lesions also may form on intestinal walls causing the lining to slough off. This form of small pox is 57% fatal in unvaccinated individuals.[1,2,8]

Hemorrhagic-type small pox is characterized by a more severe prodromal stage progressing to the development of a dusky erythema. Petechiae develop in the conjunctiva and mucous membranes. This type is highly infective and is usually fatal within 1 week. It is found most often in adults and women who are pregnant. Lastly, there is a modified form seen in previously vaccinated individuals. It has a shortened prodromal period and the rash may have both fewer lesions and be lesser in duration.[1,2,4,8]

See Table 8–5 for the various forms of small pox, their signs and symptoms, and treatment.

Complications of small pox include bacterial super-infections, skin abscesses, pneumonia, osteomyelitis, septic joint, and septicemia. Viral bronchitis and pneumonitis

TABLE 8–5 Types of Small Pox, Signs and Symptoms and Possible Treatments

TYPE	SIGNS AND SYMPTOMS	TREATMENT
Small pox	Prodromal period involving fever, nausea, vomiting, and headache followed in 2 to 3 days by the characteristic rash. Rash has a centrifugal appearance beginning on the face and moving to the extremities (unlike varicella [chicken pox], which is more central). The lesions from small pox also progress in unison from macula to vesicle, umbilicated pustula and finally scab. Patients with chicken pox will have lesions of all forms at the same time.	The effectiveness of modern antivirals remains unknown, treatment in the past was supportive in nature. Available vaccines should be given to victims, which may decrease the severity of the disease, health-care workers, other emergency providers, and potential victims surrounding the outbreak in an attempt to control the spread of the disease.
Flat-type small pox	Prodromal period involving fever, nausea, vomiting, and headache; rash develops slowly, becomes confluent, and remains flat. Rapid progression to sepsis.	Supportive care is the mainstay of treatment. This form is often fatal.
Hemorrhagic-type small pox	Severe prodromal stage progressing to the development of a dusky erythema with petechiae developing in the conjunctiva and mucous membranes.	Treatment is supportive in nature. This is also usually fatal.

may also occur. Cough is not one of the classic symptoms of small pox though it may develop. Oral secretions contain a large amount of the virus, therefore, droplets from a cough would be particularly contagious. Corneal ulcerations and keratitis also may occur and may cause blindness. This occurs most often with hemorrhagic type. Encephalitis may occur around day six to day ten when the rash is still in its papular phase.[1,2,4,8]

Treatment

There has not been a case of small pox since the development of modern antivirals so it may respond to antiviral treatment. Traditionally, treatment focuses on supportive care. Controlling nausea and vomiting may help control fluid and electrolyte imbalances during the prodromal phases. After lesions develop, the patient may still experience significant fluid losses progressing to hypovolemia and shock. Patients also may be unwilling to take oral fluids and nutrition because of discomfort from oral and pharyngeal lesions.[1,2,4,8]

In the event of a small pox outbreak, it will be necessary to use the vaccine that is currently available and stockpiled. However, this brings its own risks. Adverse outcomes from

Evidence for Practice

The rash of small pox begins on the face and spreads to the extremities; it is centrifugal in appearance unlike chicken pox, which is central. The central rash of chicken pox begins on the trunk and is concentrated there. Small pox will show a rash in which all lesions pass though various stages at the same time, whereas chicken pox will show a rash with lesions varying from early maculopapular lesions, vesicles, and scabbed-over lesions all at the same time. Chicken pox ceases to be contagious when scabbed over whereas small pox will remain contagious while lesions are present.

Any case of small pox would be devastating as a result of the lack of immunity in the world's population. This lack of immunity would allow the disease to spread rapidly and cause significant morbidity and mortality.

the vaccine are relatively rare and very rare for individuals who have previously been vaccinated, but may be serious.[12] These complications are significantly less of a concern than the disease itself. The complications of most concern follow:[4]

- **Progressive Vaccinia.** Progressive vaccinia is a progression of the lesion formed at the site of the vaccination. If the site does not heal and continues to expand beyond 15 days, progressive vaccinia should be considered. Those most at risk are those individuals who are immune suppressed by defects in their cell-mediated immune system or who are on large doses of steroids or chemotherapeutics. Areas of painless necrosis may develop at other sites on the body. The patient develops a viremia and is infective. Treatment is supportive, rarely includes surgical intervention, and may include vaccinia immune globulin (VIG) **(see Fig. 8–7).**

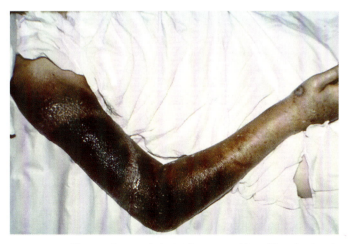

FIGURE 8–7. This 1962 photograph depicted a 70-year-old Cardiff, Wales, female smallpox patient who had received a smallpox vaccination and subsequently developed a severe reaction to the vaccine known as "vaccinia necrosum." These reactions require immediate medical attention. Progressive vaccinia (or vaccinia necrosum) is an ongoing infection of skin with tissue destruction frequently leading to death. *Photo courtesy of the Public Health Images Library, CDC.*

- **Eczema Vaccination.** Eczema vaccination affects individuals with a history of or currently active eczema (atopic dermatitis). A generalized or localized papular, pustular, or vesicular rash forms. Although the rash may form where previous eczema outbreaks have occurred, it can develop anywhere on the body. Individuals will develop fever, general malaise, and lymphadenopathy. As with progressive vaccinia, treatment includes VIG, monitoring fluid and electrolyte balance, and skin care. These patients are infectious.

- **Generalized Vaccinia.** Generalized vaccinia is a generalized macular, papular, or vesicular rash that may resemble and follow the course of the original vaccination lesion. Other than occasional fever, the patient is not symptomatic. Treatment consists of nonsteroidal anti-inflammatory drugs and antipruritics. The lesions may contain live virus. Even so, these patients are usually treated on an outpatient basis.

- **Post-Vaccination Encephalomyelitis and Post-Vaccination Encephalopathy.** The etiology of these two complications remains somewhat unclear. Post-vaccination encephalomyelitis occurs in children around 2 years of age. It is believed to be an autoimmune response. Similar to other encephalitides there is perivenous inflammation and demyelination. Cerebral spinal fluid pressure may be elevated, but is otherwise normal. Symptoms include fever, headache, vomiting, confusion, delirium, restlessness, drowsiness, lethargy, seizures, and coma. Post-vaccination encephalopathy may develop in children younger than 2 years of age. There is generalized cerebral edema, lymphocytic meningeal infiltration, ganglion degeneration, and perivascular hemorrhages. Symptoms are similar to post-vaccination encephalomyelitis with hemiplegia and aphasia. Diagnosis is difficult because no laboratory or radiological studies can differentiate these from other encephalopathies. Treatment is supportive including possible admission to an intensive care unit and anticonvulsive therapy.

- **Fetal Vaccinia.** Fetal vaccinia manifests when vaccination occurs during pregnancy. It also may occur if vaccination takes place shortly before conception. Skin lesions and problems with organ development often cause early or premature labor. Fetal or neonatal death often occurs.

- **Accidental Infection.** Accidental infection occurs when the live virus from a vaccinated individual is transferred to another part of the body. Of most concern are the eyes. Ocular vaccinia may cause blepharitis, conjunctivitis, keratitis, iritis, or any combination of these. This may result in permanent loss of or changes in vision; all cases of ocular vaccinia should be treated and followed by ophthalmology. Treatment with ocular antiviral may show promise but tests are not conclusive. Vaccinia immune globin (VIG) may be used with severe disease; however, there has been evidence linking VIG to worsened corneal scarring when these lesions were present.

- **Cardiac Concerns.** There are reports of cardiac complications following small pox vaccination. Ischemia, arrhythmias, and myopericarditis have been reported. Of these complications, myopericarditis is most common. The typical symptoms included dyspnea, palpitations, EKG changes, and cardiac enzyme elevation. During the 2003 vaccination of military and civilian health-care workers, 1 in 7000 civilian and 1 in 12,000 military personnel developed cardiac complications; all recovered.

See Table 8–6 for a listing of complications of the small pox vaccine.

Small pox remains a significant threat as a terrorist weapon. There is little or no immunity in the general population of the world. Stockpiles of the virus remain in both the United States and the former Soviet Union; a far smaller stockpile of the vaccine exists. In an aerosolized form, the virus could infect large numbers of people who would not be diagnosed for several days. This lag between infection and diagnosis would allow many victims to travel outside the initially targeted area. Given that most physicians and practitioners have never seen an actual case of small pox, it is probable that diagnosis would be slow and possibly misdiagnosed.

TABLE 8–6   Complications of Small Pox Vaccine With Signs and Symptoms

COMPLICATIONS OF SMALL POX VACCINE	SIGNS AND SYMPTOMS
Progressive vaccinia	Progression of the lesion formed at the site of the vaccination for longer than 15 days.
Eczema vaccination	Generalized or localized papular, pustular, or vesicular rash forms usually where previous eczema outbreaks have occurred, may develop anywhere on the body.
Generalized vaccinia	Generalized macular, papular, or vesicular rash that may resemble and follow the course of the original vaccination lesion.
Post-vaccination encephalomyelitis and post-vaccination encephalopathy	Children 2 years of age: Fever, headache, vomiting, confusion, delirium, restlessness, drowsiness, lethargy, seizures, and coma; similar to other encephalopathies.
Fetal vaccinia	Vaccination occurs during any of the trimesters of pregnancy or shortly before conception. May cause premature labor and fetal or neonatal death.
Accidental infection	Live virus from a vaccinated individual is transferred to another part of the body. Of most concern is the eyes. Ocular vaccinia may cause blepharitis, conjunctivitis, keratitis, or iritis.
Cardiac concerns	Ischemia, arrhythmias, and myopericarditis.

The vaccine used to protect health-care workers, the military, and those in proximity to the outbreak (in efforts to contain the outbreak) is limited and may cause significant, possibly fatal complications. Given these complications and limitations, small pox in the hands of a terrorist would be a deadly weapon of terror worldwide.[1,2,4,8]

Viral Hemorrhagic Fever

Viral hemorrhagic fever (VHF) is caused by groups of viruses with variations on a common presentation. The most significant outbreaks appear to have occurred in or as a result of someone or something traveling from Africa. As bioterrorist agents, there are four types of viruses which are of concern: Filoviridae, Arenaviridae, Bunyaviridae, and Flaviviridae. Filoviridae include Ebola and Marburg viruses. Arenaviridae include Lassa fever virus and a group of New World viruses such as Junin virus, Machupo virus, and Sabia virus. The Bunyaviridae group includes Rift Valley fever virus and Hantaviruses. Finally, Flaviviridae group includes yellow fever, dengue fever, and others.[2,4,8,13]

Transmission and Signs and Symptoms

The typical common presentation is hemorrhagic manifestations, maculopapular rash, rapidly progressive disease leading to shock, and death in 1 week. Ebola and Marburg are transmitted person to person through direct contact with blood, tissue, or secretions. Percutaneous contaminated needle sticks appear to be particularly effective in transmitting the disease. Direct contact with contaminated fingers to eyes and mucous membranes also is effective. The natural reservoir of the virus is unknown[2,4,8,13] **(see Fig. 8–8).**

Lassa fever and New World adenoviruses viruses also are transmitted person to person via direct contact with blood and bodily secretions. It is not, however, transmitted via droplet through the respiratory system. The natural reservoir for these viruses is rodents. Direct contact with open wounds, inhalation of particles of urine or feces, or ingestion of food contaminated with infected rodent waste is the normal route of infection for humans.[2,4,8,13]

Bunyaviridae viruses cause Rift Valley fever (RVF), Crimean Congo hemorrhagic fever (CCHF), and Hantavirus infection. They are transmitted through both rodent and insect vectors; including ticks and mosquitoes or direct contact with

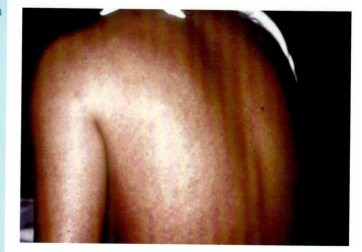

FIGURE 8–8. This posterior-oblique view of the back of a female with Marburg virus disease (case #2), shows a measles-like rash, a usual symptom of this viral illness. This patient was hospitalized in Johannesburg, South Africa, 1975. This type of maculopapular rash, which can appear on patients with Marburg virus disease around the fifth day after the onset of symptoms, usually appears on the patient's chest, back, and stomach. This patient's skin blanched under pressure, which is a common characteristic of a Marburg virus rash. Treatment is supportive, including fluids and symptom relief. *Photo courtesy of the Public Health Images Library, CDC.*

contaminated tissue or inhalation of the virus from carcasses. RVF is not transmitted human to human whereas CCHF has been shown to infect health-care workers. Hantavirus has, in the past, been considered a significant threat as a bioterrorist weapon like RVF and CCHF, but that is no longer the case. Hantavirus manifests as either a pulmonary syndrome or hemorrhagic with renal failure and has a high mortality but it is not easily weaponized and is hard to produce in large quantities. Also it is not easily transmitted and may be easily prevented and treated.[2,4,8,13]

Flaviviridae viruses cause yellow fever, dengue fever, and other VHFs. Of these, dengue fever is considered a significant threat as a bioterrorist weapon. No human-to-human contact has been reported. Transmission to humans is through mosquito bites[2,4,8,13] **(see Table 8–7).**

TABLE 8–7 Viruses Associated With Viral Hemorrhagic Fever, How They Are Spread and Their Reservoirs

VIRUS	DISEASE	HOW DISEASE IS SPREAD	VECTOR
Filoviridae	Ebola and Marburg	Human-to-human contact with blood, tissue, and secretions. Percutaneous needle stick particularly effective.	Reservoir unknown
Arenaviridae	Lassa fever, Junin, Machupo, and Sabia fevers	Blood and direct human-to-human contact; not spread through respiratory secretions.	Reservoir rodents
Bunyaviridae	Rift Valley and Hanta viruses	Human-to-human contact.	Reservoir both rodent and insect
Flaviviridae	Yellow and dengue fevers	Spread through insect vector. Not spread through human-to-human contact	Reservoir mosquitoes
Treatment	Strict isolation of victims. Supportive care for all VHFs. Fever control, fluid and electrolyte balance, and pain control.		

Treatment

VHF presents with acute fever, hypotension, petechiae, hemorrhage, conjunctival infection, flushing, edema, malaise, prostration, myalgias, arthralgias, rash, headache, nausea, vomiting, diarrhea, and abdominal pain. Shock, pulmonary issues, neurological, and hematopoietic concerns follow. Fatality rates range from as low as 1% with RVF to as high as 50% with Hantavirus. Most range from 20% to 35%. Treatment is supportive. Fluid and electrolyte balance may be difficult to maintain. Both hypotension and pulmonary edema may develop. Vasopressors may be necessary. Anticoagulants, nonsteroidal anti-inflammatory drugs (NSAIDs), and intramuscular injections should be avoided.[2,4,8,13]

Consider VHF for anyone with fever, maculopapular rash, or signs of hemorrhage without cough, or nasal congestion who has traveled to or is from an area where VHF is endemic, had direct contact with infected tissue or blood, or worked in a laboratory dealing with any of these viruses. Any victims of VHF who have not traveled within 3 weeks to endemic areas, not worked with infected tissue or virus in a laboratory should raise the suspicion of a bioterrorist attack. Laboratory confirmation is done in conjunction with public health and the CDC. Ribavirin may be effective in treating VHF. An experimental vaccine for Ebola and other forms of VHF may be available. The vaccine is rapid acting making it possible to vaccinate populations surrounding an outbreak, thereby containing it.[2,8,13,14]

VHFs pose a significant threat to the general population. Natural outbreaks are limited to Africa or caused by contact with people or animals from Africa. They are generally very contagious with significant morbidity and mortality. Treatment is difficult with supportive care the only choice.[4,13]

Botulism

The toxin created by the bacteria *Clostridium botulinum* is the most toxic substance known to man. It is 15,000 to 100,000 times more toxic than VX and sarin nerve agents. *C. botulinum* is commonly found in the environment with most outbreaks resulting from poor canning techniques. Botulinum toxin is approved by the Food and Drug Administration (FDA) for treatment of neuromuscular disorders such as strabismus or torticollis. It also is used off-label cosmetically for wrinkles or for headaches, low back pain, stroke, achalasia, or dystonias. It is important to note that the preparation used in these instances is diluted to 0.3% to 0.005% of the lethal oral or inhalation dose.[2,4]

Botulism has four human natural forms; food-borne, wound, infantile, and intestinal. Food-borne botulism is a result of eating improperly canned or prepared foods. Both canned meats and garden foods are susceptible. Wound botulism results from wounds contaminated with *C. botulinum*. It then grows in the anaerobic environment and releases the toxin. Infantile botulism occurs with the endogenous production of the bacteria in the intestines of an infant after the ingestion of *C. botulinum* spores. Intestinal botulism is similar, but occurs in children or adults when no other source can be identified. Inhalational botulism is a fifth type. It does not occur naturally and is caused by the inhalation of the toxin. It should always be considered an intentional act or accidental laboratory exposure[2,4] **(see Fig. 8–9).**

Botulism bacteria have four distinctly different genetic types that produce seven distinct toxins: A, B, C_1, D, E, F, and G.

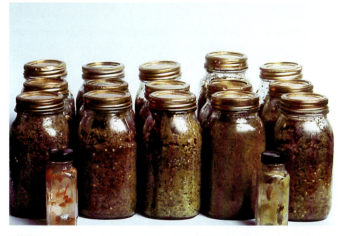

FIGURE 8–9. These are jars of contaminated Jalapeño peppers involved in an outbreak of botulism in Pontiac, Michigan, April, 1977. The bacterium *C. botulinum* produces a nerve toxin that causes the rare but serious paralytic illness botulism. There are seven types of botulism toxin designated by the letters A through G; only types A, B, E, and F cause illness in humans. Multiple cases of botulism without a common food source should be suspicious for respiratory botulism, which would be considered a terrorist attack. *Photo courtesy of the Public Health Images Library, CDC.*

Botulism, *continued*

There is a type C_2 that is a cytotoxin, not a neurotoxin. Of these, types A, B, and E primarily affect humans whereas types C_1 and D affect mammals or birds. Type A toxin is primarily found west of the Mississippi River; type B is found east of the Mississippi River. Type E toxin is found in the Great Lakes region, Pacific Northwest, and Alaska and is often found associated with fish products. A trivalent antitoxin, covering toxins A, B, and E, is available through Public Health departments and the CDC. The antitoxin must match the toxin to be of any value. If a toxin other than A, B, or E is suspected, as would be possible in the event of an intentional release, the military has an A, B, C, D, E, F, G antitoxin. Time concerns, the potential number of victims, and the limited supply mean that antitoxin use in the event of a mass casualty contamination may be somewhat limited.[2,4]

Signs and Symptoms

The botulism toxin blocks the release of the neurotransmitter acetylcholine. Without the release of this neurotransmitter, muscles cannot contract and a flaccid paralysis develops. Botulism is characterized by descending facial paralysis with bulbar palsies beginning with double or blurred vision, difficulty talking, and swallowing. The paralysis will continue downward to the diaphragm and extremities. The victim will be afebrile. The patient will have an intact sensorium and be alert and may not be able to respond. If fever does develop, it

WHY IS IT IMPORTANT   To Recognize Botulism Symptoms?

Numerous patients presenting afebrile with descending symmetrical paralysis and cranial nerve involvement without common food consumption should be investigated as inhalation botulism from a terrorist act. Botulism is always associated with food consumption or a dirty wound. There has never been a known incident of airborne botulism, but theoretically the toxin could be processed, aerosolized, and then sprayed over a large area. Symptoms would then occur in a large number of victims without a common food source.

is related to an opportunistic infection. Food-borne botulism begins with nausea, cramping, diarrhea, and vomiting from the tainted food; other forms do not. The botulism toxin irreversibly binds to the nerve terminal. Once there, the signs and symptoms will persist until regeneration of the axon twigs to enervate the paralyzed muscle fibers. For adults, this takes weeks to months. The severity of the symptoms of botulism can range from quite mild to so severe that the patient may appear comatose[2,4] **(see Table 8–8).**

TABLE 8–8 Botulism Toxin, Treatments, and Signs and Symptoms

TOXIN	ENDEMIC AREA	SIGNS AND SYMPTOMS	TREATMENT
Toxin A	Found west of the Mississippi in the United States.	For all forms of botulism, there is a progressive flaccid paralysis that beings with the cranial nerves and progresses downward. The victims will present with double vision and weakness of the facial muscles. This will progress downward and include the respiratory system. Throughout the progression of the disease, the victim's sensorium will remain completely intact.	Administration of Trivalent (A,B, E) antitoxin essential to halt progression of flaccid paralysis. Will not reverse any paralysis already present. Supportive care may include long-term ventilatory care. After paralyzed, the victim will require complete care until recovery, which may take months. Extensive history should be obtained to identify food source and other potential victims. If no food source is identified, inhaled botulism should be considered. This could be a laboratory accident or terrorist attack.

Continued

TABLE 8–8 Botulism Toxin, Treatments, and Signs and Symptoms—cont'd

TOXIN	ENDEMIC AREA	SIGNS AND SYMPTOMS	TREATMENT
Toxin B	Found east of the Mississippi in the United States.		Treatment same as Toxin A.
Toxin E	Found in the Great Lakes region of the United States.		Same as Toxin A.
Toxin C1 and D	Affects mammals other than humans and birds.		No treatment.
Toxin F and G	Not endemic to any areas in the United States.		If administration of Trivalent antitoxin does not halt progression of symptoms, then terrorist attack should be considered. Military has limited supply of A, B, C, D, E, F, G antitoxin available. Otherwise treatment is supportive.

Treatment

Treatment for victims of botulism is supportive and depends on the severity of symptoms. This may include ventilator support until resolution. The antitoxin should be administered as soon as possible because it only halts progression of the paralysis and cannot reverse any already present. A significant number of patients may be sensitive to the antitoxin. A skin sensitivity test should be performed before administration of the antitoxin. Those with significant flare or wheal should be desensitized before administration of the antitoxin to avoid a possible anaphylaxis reaction. The administration of antitoxin for infant botulism is questionable because it may induce a lifelong sensitivity to equine antigens. Treatment is supportive care.[2,4]

Gastric lavage and the administration of charcoal may be appropriate for food-borne botulism depending on the time between ingestion and presentation. These actions may facilitate the removal of residual toxin in the gastrointestinal tract.

An in-depth history and physical must be performed including recent travel, foods eaten, where they were eaten, and who else may have consumed them. Patients may travel a significant distance before presentation of symptoms. The disease is often misdiagnosed; therefore, it is important to contact all potential victims, include them in the investigation, and ensure proper treatment. Botulism or the suspicion of botulism is legally reportable to the local health department.[2,4]

Routine laboratory and radiological testing is of little value in the diagnosis of botulism. Lumbar puncture also may not yield definitive results. Guillain-Barré syndrome, often mistakenly diagnosed in a patient with botulism, may show normal cerebral spinal fluid early in the progression of the disease whereas botulism may show increased protein found in Guillain-Barré. The CDC and a limited number of state health departments are equipped to perform diagnostic testing for botulism. Serum, stool, gastric contents, vomitus (if available), and the suspected food should be sent if possible. Samples should be gathered before the administration of antitoxin. Contact the appropriate laboratory and public health department for directions concerning obtaining, storing, and transferring the samples. If inhalation botulism is suspected, a nasal swab should be obtained, but must be obtained within 24 hours of exposure. It is extremely important that a complete list of the patient's medications accompany the collected samples because these medications may affect some of the testing.[2,4]

Botulism toxin is the most toxic substance known. It was previously thought that it posed a threat from terrorist groups aiming to contaminate municipal water supplies. This is no longer a concern because of the susceptibility of both the bacteria and toxin to chlorination. However, mass contamination through food supplies or inhalation remains a potential threat. Treatment is limited to supportive care and a limited supply of antitoxin. This antitoxin will only halt the progression of the symptoms not reverse those already present. Any degree of paralysis present will not resolve for weeks to months.

Victims of botulism are often misdiagnosed with other neurological diseases such as Guillain-Barré syndrome, myasthenia gravis, hypothyroidism, and others, delaying much-needed treatment with antitoxin. Resources, such as ventilators, for supportive care in the event of a mass outbreak may be extremely limited and therefore devastating. As with other agents, the intentional use of botulism toxin as a terrorist weapon could result in significant morbidity and mortality.[2,4]

Summary

The specter of a biological attack or accidental release remains a significant concern today. Each of the agents discussed has the potential to cause devastating morbidity and mortality. Beyond this, an intentional release would cause considerable social disruption and panic. With incubation periods ranging from 3 to 7 days and infectivity 7 to 17 days, travel outside of the site of original infection will occur, making containment extremely difficult. The federal government through the CDC, United States Army Medical Research Institute for Infectious Diseases (USAMRIID), Department of Health and Human Services, the United States Marine Corp Chemical and Biological Incident Response Force, the Army's Technical Escort Unit (for sampling), the special Medical Augmentation Response teams, the Federal Bureau of Investigation, and the National Guard ten rapid assessment and initial response teams are all available to assist in treatment and containment of biological (and chemical) attacks or outbreaks. The initial detection response and containment must come from astute and alert health-care providers.[4,15]

Nursing, both as registered nurses and as APNs, is a significant part of the health-care workforce and should remain familiar with the signs, symptoms, and treatment regimens for these agents. The specter of terrorist attack or accidental outbreak remains real and should be considered when developing undergraduate curriculum and continuing education programs. In spite of the rare presentation of these diseases, nursing must remain aware of their potential and prepare for them.

Nursing administration should facilitate this by looking for graduate nurses from programs that provide this education. They also should stress disaster education, including biological agents, as part of the competencies established for their institution. Gathering and disseminating this information when an outbreak is suspected will not provide a working knowledge or level of skill required to respond in a crisis.

Lastly, research is needed regarding nursing and medical preparations and response to these agents. They are rare in the United States, but may be endemic to other parts of the world. Analysis of nursing and medical care from these areas and historical data to provide insights into best practices may be essential to treat and contain outbreaks in the future.

REFERENCES

1. O'Connell KP, Menuey BC, Foster D. Issues in preparedness for biologic terrorism: a perspective for critical care nursing. *AACN Clinical Issues.* 2002;13(3):452–469.
2. Varkey P, Poland GA, Cockerill FR, Smith TF, Hagen PT. Confronting bioterrorism: physicians on the front line.[see comment]. *Mayo Clinic Proceedings.* 2002;77(7):661–672.
3. Crupi RS, Asnis DS, Lee CC, Santucci T, Marino MJ, Flanz BJ. Meeting the challenge of bioterrorism: lessons learned from West Nile virus and anthrax. *American Journal of Emergency Medicine.* 2003;21(1):77–79.
4. Keyes DC ed. *Medical Response to Terrorism.* Philadelphia, PA: Lippincott Williams & Wilkins; 2005, 449.
5. Altman GB. Bioterrorism's invisible threats: heightened awareness will help nurses identify real and suspected bioterrorism. *Nursing Management.* 2002;33(1):43.

6. Greenfield RA, Drevets DA, Machado LJ, Coskuhl GW, Bronze MS. Bacterial pathogens as biological weapons and agents of bioterrorism. *American Journal of the Medical Sciences.* 2002;323(6):299–315.

7. Centers for Disease Control and Prevention. Bioterrorism alleging use of anthrax and interim guidelines for management—United States, 1998. *MMWR—Morbidity & Mortality Weekly Report.* 1999;48(4):69–74.

8. Cunha BA. Anthrax, tularemia, plague, Ebola or smallpox as agents of bioterrorism: recognition in the emergency room. *Clinical Microbiology and Infection.* 2002;8(8):489–503.

9. Celia F. Cutaneous anthrax: an overview. *Dermatology Nursing.* 2002;14(2):89–92.

10. Guffey MB, Dalzell A, Kelly Dr, Cassady KA. Ulceroglandular tularemia in a nonendemic area. *Southern Medical Journal.* 2007;100(3):304–308.

11. Johansson A, Berglund L, Gothefors L, Sjöstedt A, Tärnvik A. Ciprofloxacin for treatment of tularemia in children. *Pediatric Infectious Disease Journal.* 2000;19(5): 449–453.

12. Cohen HW, Gould RM, Sidel VW. the pitfalls of bioterrorism preparedness: the anthrax and smallpox experiences. *American Journal of Public Health.* 2004;94(10):1667–1671.

13. Borio L, Inglesby T, Peters CJ, et al. Hemorrhagic fever viruses as biological weapons: medical and public health management. *JAMA.* 2002;287(18):2391–2405.

14. Baize S, Marianneau P, Georges-Courbot MC, Deubel V. Recent advances in vaccines against viral haemorrhagic fevers. *Current Opinion in Infectious Diseases.* 2001;14(5):513–518.

15. Clawson A, Menachemi N, Beitsch L, Brooks RG. Are community health centers prepared for bioterrorism? *Biosecurity and Bioterrorism.* 2006;4(1): 55–63.

Chemical Agents

Introduction

Nursing and other health-care providers need to be aware of the potentially devastating consequences of chemical disasters. Incidents caused by many of the agents covered in this chapter are extremely rare; however, other chemicals discussed here are common and could cause serious concerns from an accidental or intentional release. There has never been a release of nerve agents or vesicants within the United States but they have been used in recent history by terrorist groups and other countries. Chemicals of a similar nature continue to be available commercially for pest control and for use in manufacturing processes. As health-care providers, nurses and advanced practice nurses (APNs) need to be aware of the signs, symptoms, and treatment protocols of these rare chemicals and also more common chemicals such as cyanide or chlorine. Large releases could cause victims to present to local hospitals in overwhelming numbers.

Nursing administration should be concerned with providing the appropriate equipment and training for decontamination. Studies have shown that victims will bypass triage and decontamination at the scene of the incident and present directly to the hospital for treatment. If allowed to enter the emergency department before decontamination, all or part of the area becomes unusable by other patients. Administration should advocate for construction designs or add on equipment to meet these needs. Continuing education needs of the medical and nursing staff should provide the information and training to meet the competencies required to care for victims of chemical releases. Applicants from graduate and undergraduate programs that provide the training within their curriculums should be given priority.

Graduate and undergraduate programs should include information concerning chemical incidents, signs, symptoms, and treatment along with other disaster education within their curriculum. It is important that students come away from these programs understanding the importance of this information regardless of the rarity of presentation. Untrained health-care personnel cannot effectively respond to these or other disasters without previous training and competence.

Chemical Incidents

Chemical incidents can be broadly classified in two ways: intentional and unintentional. Treatment and preparation varies significantly according to the agent and the involvement of law enforcement. Intentional incidents are defined as criminal acts of terrorism or sabotage causing the release of toxic chemicals into the environment and causing harm to both the environment and humans. Unintentional incidents have the same results; however, the release is accidental.

An extremely important aspect of the risk assessment performed by an organization or community is the examination of the potential for intentional or unintentional chemical incidents. Large metropolitan areas or locations prone to large gatherings of people or areas of strategic importance may be at risk for both intentional and unintentional incidents. However, unintentional incidents are possible anywhere there is chemical

WHY IS IT IMPORTANT To Be Prepared?

Although chemical incidents are somewhat rare, all areas where significant industry or transportation infrastructure exist and population centers with water treatment facilities are potentially at risk for a chemical incident. Adequate preparation including risk assessment, development of treatment protocols for nursing, nurse practitioners, and physicians are essential for prompt effective treatment.

manufacturing, transportation infrastructure, or water treatment facilities. Even very rural areas with drinking or waste water treatment facilities store and use chlorine. The highway and rail systems traverse both highly developed and sparsely populated areas making virtually any place a potential site for a chemical incident. It is imperative that communities and institutions be prepared to respond.[1-3] The Joint Commission (TJC), several government agencies, and specific laws require health-care facilities to have adequate disaster planning, equipment, and training to provide care in response to a chemical incident.[2]

Preparation and Response

It is beyond the scope of this book to cover all of the concerns of community preparation and response. Chemical and biological events requiring containment, isolation, and decontamination are complex and can be very expensive; however, communities and institutions must be prepared to both decontaminate victims and contain the toxic agent. Every chemical event must be contained and decontamination takes place at the scene of the incident. This is vital to control the spread of the toxin and prevent further contamination particularly of treatment facilities. This certainly places the initial and perhaps most significant response in the hands of the community emergency response organizations.[1,2,4,5]

The primary response to a chemical incident falls to industrial hazardous material teams and local fire and emergency services. Responsibilities include containment of the incident, containment of the toxic agent, and decontamination of both the environment and victims.[3,6,7] This requires a significant investment in finances and training. Training must be ongoing; at the very least every 2 years, if not yearly. Equipment should include decontamination shelters, shower facilities, the availability of large quantities of water and low-pressure capabilities, and personal protective equipment (PPE). PPE provides protection against chemical or radioactive agents with protection ranging from level

D, minimal work uniforms such as scrubs, to level A, completely sealed from particulates, vapors, and liquids with a self-contained source of air.[1–5,8]

Health-care institutions such as hospitals and possibly clinics must also be prepared to contain and decontaminate victims and equipment from a chemical event. It has been shown that victims will be transported, by either private or emergency vehicles, to treatment facilities before the true cause is known. Any vehicle, public or private, or any treatment area in which a victim may have been, should now be considered contaminated. Examination of past events indicates that Good Samaritans may offer to transport victims from events to treatment facilities, potentially contaminating themselves and their vehicles. It has also been evident from past events that victims may not wait for decontamination and treatment at the scene, but proceed directly to treatment facilities, further contaminating vehicles and treatment areas. Hospitals must be made aware of events with possible contamination as soon as possible. They in turn must be prepared to control and decontaminate victims before they enter treatment areas.[1–5] In 1995, in an incident in Tokyo, Japan when the Aum Shinriko released sarin in subways during rush hour, 85% of the victims reported directly to the nearest health-care facility bypassing emergency medical services (EMS) and decontamination.[9] Typically, there is a significant amount of time necessary before victims can begin to be treated at the scene. Local fire and EMS need to be notified; respond; establish zones

WHY IS IT IMPORTANT **To Remain Vigilant?**

Decontamination must occur at the scene; however, evidence has shown that victims will bypass treatment at the scene and present directly to a hospital for decontamination and treatment. This means that large numbers of contaminated victims will present directly to the emergency department for treatment. Nursing must be vigilant for potential victims and hospitals must be prepared to decontaminate victims outside the main treatment area to prevent further spread.

of contamination, cold, warm, and hot zones; assemble the decontamination equipment; triage; and decontaminate the victims. Victims may simply leave before directed to stay or may not be willing to wait for decontamination at the scene.

Security

Security issues are covered extensively in another section of this book; however, they take on significant importance under these circumstances. Potentially large numbers of vehicles and people will be presenting to the institution. Victims, vehicles, and equipment must be isolated until decontaminated; this may extend to personal vehicles. Controlling the flow of contaminated and potentially contaminated victims is extremely important. Worried unaffected individuals, those who are probably not contaminated but are worried that they are, may present in large numbers. Family of victims will arrive and want to be with their loved ones. Local and perhaps national media may arrive. In the midst of all of this potential confusion, it is important to prevent the spread of contamination to uncontaminated areas. Decontamination requires the victim to remove all clothing and valuables. Security must protect the dignity and privacy of these victims.[1–3,5]

Protective Equipment

All personnel coming in contact with contaminated vehicles, equipment, or victims must wear protective equipment **(see Fig. 9–1)**. Protective equipment falls into four categories: A, B, C, and D, with D offering the least protection and A the most:[1,2,4,5,8]

- **Level A** level of protection is a vinyl sealed suit with completely self-contained air supply. No personnel should work alone dressed in level C through A suits for personal safety concerns.
- **Level B** protective equipment is similar to Class C except that there is a self-contained air supply for use if necessary.
- **Level C** equipment was developed specifically for use in the hospital setting. It consists of a Tyvec suit, rubber boots, and

doubled rubber gloves all sealed with duct tape. A powered air-purifying respirator (PAPR) hood with continuous filtered respirator provides fresh air within the hood. This level of protection should be used in a situation in which the agent is known and this level of protection is sufficient for the agent.

- **Level D** equipment or clothing is simply a required uniform such as scrubs or maintenance uniforms.

Decontamination

Decontamination is usually accomplished using large amounts of water under low pressure with gentle scrubbing with soap and a soft brush if necessary and is carried out in a portable or permanent shower.[1,2,4–8]

- Those very rare chemicals that react with water, such as metallic sodium, should be removed with forceps and stored in oil.

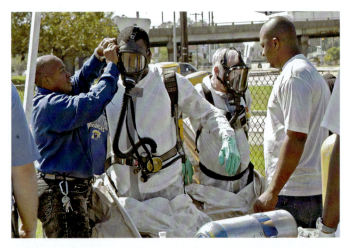

FIGURE 9–1. Baton Rouge, Louisiana, October 9, 2005. A HAZMAT instructor (left) adjusts the respirator mask being used by one of two area Emergency Medical Technician team members who are preparing to respond to a simulated rescue operation of a chemical spill. All first responders cleaning up the toxic conditions caused by Hurricanes Katrina and Rita have undergone similar training. *Source: Win Henderson/FEMA.*

- Moisture on the skin and in the air also may cause the chemical to react harming the victim more. Therefore, remove the contaminant as quickly as possible, which may involve the use of large quantities of water even with those reactive chemicals.
- Contaminated clothing should be removed; this may remove as much as 80% of the contamination.
- Grossly contaminated dust should be gently brushed from the victims and large amounts of water under low pressure used to remove any further contamination.
- Jewelry, if at all possible, should be removed and the skin beneath cleansed.
- Victims who are unable to walk or who are strapped to a backboard will require personnel to remove their clothing and jewelry and wash the patient using low-pressure hoses. Victim's privacy should be maintained as much as possible without further endangering them.

The victim's eyes and lungs may require special attention.

- Eyes may have to be anesthetized with a topical anesthetic and flushed with a Morgan lens and large amounts of a sterile, neutral solution such as normal saline.
- Eyes should be flushed until symptoms are gone or the eye returns to a normal pH.
- The respiratory system may be significantly affected by inhaled agents and may be compromised.
- Other agents may be absorbed through the skin and affect oxygen carrying capacity or the ability of the lungs to exchange gases. Treatment includes oxygen and possible intubation to assist patient respiration.

Water used in the decontamination process should be collected if at all possible and disposed of through appropriate hazardous material agencies. When this is not possible because of large quantity of water or lack of adequate containment facilities, it may be possible to suspend local and national pollution laws and dispose of the run off through the sewer system. All efforts should be made to contact the local water authority and notify them of the incident.

Patient belongings should be placed in plastic bags for disposal or decontamination. Each bag should be marked with the patient's name or identification number listed on the patient's disaster tag. As much as possible, care should be taken to not lose or confuse victim belongings. Special care should be taken with jewelry, wallets, and other valuables. Valuables should remain with the victim if at all possible. Advice and assistance with possible decontamination of valuables should be provided before the patient is released. Some valuables or important papers may have to be disposed of if decontamination is impossible.[1,5,8]

After initial gross decontamination, the victim should be assessed for injuries, signs and symptoms related to the contaminating agent, and for further needs including social and psychological concerns. Depending on the nature of the event and the agent, there may be a significant number of contaminated and affected patients requiring further significant treatment or there may be a large number of worried patients requiring more assurance than treatment. In a large-scale event, there will be both.[1,4,5,8]

Classification of Chemical Agents

Discussion of agents/chemicals, in general, can be organized in three classes.

- **Class I** chemicals are those with no use in commercial manufacturing and have a significant possibility for use as chemical weapons. Examples of these would be mustard agents or VX, a nerve agent.
- **Class II** chemicals are those with some commercial application, but also have significant possible use as a chemical weapon. This class would include chlorine or phosgene.
- **Class III** chemicals are those of limited use as chemical weapons. It is important to note that these agents may still be extremely toxic to humans and the environment or pose long-term health hazards requiring significant action on the part of local hazard material teams in case of a spill.

Class I Agents

Class I chemicals have no use other than as terrorist agents and weapons of mass destruction. They include mustard gas and nerve agents; of these, nerve agents are the most toxic and deadly. Nerve agents are commonly called nerve gas, though they are liquids. They trace their origins to industrial World War II Germany and were originally developed as insecticides. They are most effective when inhaled; however, they can be absorbed through the skin. Mustard is a gas that causes sores and lesions on the skin and eventual asphyxiation. Often death occurs as a result of continued exposure from contaminated clothing. **See Table 9–1** for a listing of lethal concentrations and topical doses of nerve agents.

Nerve Agents

Nerve agents were developed first as insecticides in Germany around 1936 as organophosphates. Tabun was first developed with sarin following. At the end of World War II, the manufacturing facility was dismantled and moved to the Soviet Union. The United States and the Soviet Union were very active in the continued development of nerve agents. After the development of sarin, soman and, finally, VX were developed.[9]

TABLE 9–1 Lethal Concentrations of Topical Doses of Nerve Agents			
NERVE AGENT	FORM	LETHAL CONCENTRATION	LETHAL TOPICAL DOSE
Tabun	Volatile	400 mg/min/m³	1000 mg
Sarin	Volatile	100 mg/min/m³	1700 mg
Soman	Volatile	50 mg/min/m³	100 mg
VX	Oily liquid	10 mg/min/m³	10 mg

Tabun, sarin, and soman are considered volatile agents whereas VX is an oily liquid. The lethality of these agents is measured as LCt_{50}; that is, the dose would kill 50% of unprotected humans exposed for 1 minute in a concentration per cubic meter. Tabun has an LCt_{50} of 400 mg/min/m³, sarin 100 mg/min/m³, soman 50 mg/min/m³, and VX 10 mg/min/m³. The volatility of the agents, that is how much will **off-gas,** that is, become a gas at a given temperature, must also be considered. The volatility of each agent at 25°C is significantly more than a lethal dose. At most environmental temperatures, these agents will place enough chemical into the atmosphere to be lethal. All of the agents are heavier than air and therefore will not dissipate without a significant wind and in an enclosed area, they will accumulate at ground level. Contact with a small amount of liquid is also lethal. Topical lethal doses for each agent is: tabun 1000 mg, sarin 1700 mg, soman 100 mg, and VX 10 mg.[6,7,10,11]

Signs and Symptoms

Nerve agents are the most lethal of chemical agents. They act to inhibit acetylcholinesterase thereby blocking the breakdown of acetylcholine, causing its buildup and sending the victim into a cholinergic crisis, which causes the signs and symptoms. Ganglionic, nicotinic, and cholinergic excesses result in tachycardia, hypertension, mydriasis, and salivation, lacrimation, urination, diaphoresis, deification, GI motility, and emesis (SLUDGE). Another acronym used is DUMBELS, (diarrhea, urination, miosis, bronchoconstriction, bronchorrhea, emesis, lacrimation, and salivation) **(see Table 9–2).** Local effects from topical exposure also cause muscle fasciculations. Vapors will cause an increase in eye and respiratory symptoms. Generalized weakness and seizures follow; leading to eventual flaccid paralysis, respiratory failure, and death.[6,7,10,11]

The seizures caused by these agents do not originate from one focus in the brain as common seizures do. Seizures are caused by both the agent and a buildup of acylcholine throughout the brain so that seizures originate from the whole brain. The seizures also are tied to glutamate, which is triggered by the seizure activity and perpetuates the

TABLE 9–2　Signs and Symptoms of Nerve Agents and Organophosphates

S	Salivation	D	Diarrhea
L	Lacrimation	U	Urination
U	Urination	M	Miosis
D	Diaphoresis	B	Bronchospasm & Bronchorrhea
G	GI Motility	E	Emesis
E	Emesis	L	Lacrimation
		S	Salivation

Evidence for Practice

Seizures as a result of exposure to nerve agents do not originate in one focus within the brain but involve the whole brain and only respond to benzodiazepines. Other antiseizure medications such as Dilantin have no effect in controlling seizure activity. It also is extremely important to note that seizure activity may continue after flaccid paralysis has set in. This continued seizure activity is extremely damaging to the brain. Rhythmic movement of the victim's eyes may indicate that the victim is still seizing.

seizure, leading to status epilepticus, which occurs within 30 to 60 minutes of exposure.

There may be no typical seizure activity after the victim develops flaccid paralysis. The seizures may only manifest by EEG or small rhythmic movements of the victim's eyes. The victim may also be tachycardic, hypertensive, and develop apnea. This type of seizure may be differentiated from a head injury that manifests as hypertension, bradycardia, and irregular breathing patterns. If seizure activity is suspected, it must be treated. Seizure activity takes an enormous amount of energy. After the body has used up all available adenosine triphosphate (ATP), it reverts to anaerobic energy production leading to a buildup of lactic acid. The seizure activity, the buildup of lactic acid, and the agent itself all will cause brain injury, long-term effects, or death.[6,7,10,11]

Long-term effects of exposure to nerve agents include short-term memory loss (long-term memory is not affected), insomnia, headaches, blurred vision (especially at night), anxiety, decreases in ability to concentrate, confusion, short temper, runny nose, and chest tightness. These affects may last weeks to months and may be mild to moderate in intensity.

Treatment

If the agent is known, Level B or C protective equipment should be worn for the decontamination process. If the agent is unknown, Level A protective equipment should be used. Once decontamination has been completed, standard precautions include Level D protective equipment and standard universal precautions.

Treatment of nerve agents involves both pretreatment, when possible, and treatment of symptoms after exposure. Topical agents may be used to minimize absorption of the nerve agent. Pretreatment also involves the use of physostigmine bromide. Physostigmine bromide, unlike nerve agents, reversibly blocks acetylcholinesterase; nerve agents bind permanently. After a person is exposed to the nerve agent, the reversible bond with physostigmine bromide blocks a portion of the affects and then releases from the neuron resulting in the return of a portion of normal function. The victim will still be sick, both before and after the exposure to the agent, but with a lesser severity. Pretreatment is essential for some agents such as soman, which work so quickly there may not be time to treat with atropine and other supportive agents. There also is research into a bioscavenger protein that would inactivate the nerve agent.[6,7,10,11]

Treatment of victims after exposure involves treatment of symptoms with atropine and dioxime mytupan. These medications work on the peripheral effects of the nerve agent but offer no treatment for the central nervous system and the treatment of seizures. Seizure activity has been traditionally treated in the field with diazepam because of ease of intramuscular injection. Most research and development of treatment has been from the military. A concern about diazepam as an intramuscular injection has been erratic up take. In the hospital setting and in the field through emergency medical services, the ability of IV access significantly improves treatment options. Any benzodiazepine may be used to treat seizure activity with varying degrees of effectiveness. It is important to note that other antiseizure agents, such as phenytoin, are ineffective in treating seizures caused by nerve agents.[6,7,10,11]

Atropine acts to treat central and systemic muscarinic effects. It alleviates bronchospasm. The dose should begin at 1 to 3 mg but may require significantly more. The endpoint dose should be judged by the decrease in bronchospasm, bronchosecretions, and the subsequent decrease in airway resistance. The dose may be as much as 5 to 15 mg in the case of nerve agents or several grams in the case of organophosphate insecticides.[10,11]

Oximes such as pralidoxime or obidoxime work by reactivating acetylcholinesterase. These medications must be used before the agent ages; that is, forms a permanent bond. Each agent ages at a different rate ranging from seconds to days. Sarin ages in 5 to 12 hours, whereas soman is aged in 40 seconds to 10 minutes. VX ages in 50 to 60 hours, more than 2 days. Tabun is aged in 46 hours. Once the agents have aged, the bond is permanent and requires enzyme or cellular replacement. Pralidoxime chloride (2PAMCl) or mesylate (P25) are dosed at 30 mg/kg, given over 30 minutes every 4 to 6 hours. Preferable route is IV but may be administered intramuscularly. Treatment should continue until the active metabolite of the agent is undetectable. **Table 9–3** shows aging times of nerve agents.[6,7,10,11] The long-term effect of nerve agents may be treated symptomatically with scopolamine, Topamax (not FDA approved for this treatment at the time of publication, reader should check for the most current information), or treatments similar to those for post-traumatic stress syndrome.

Testing for the continued presence and effects of nerve agents may be accomplished through examination of red blood

TABLE 9–3	Aging Times of Nerve Agents
AGENT	AGING TIME*
Sarin	5 to 12 hours
Soman	40 seconds to 10 minutes
Tabun	46 hours
VX	50 to 60 hours

*After the agent is "aged" the bond is permanent.

cells (RBCs). Acetylcholinesterase does not act as a neurotransmitter in RBCs, it is, however, present and may be measured as RBC-ChE or BChE. BChE correlates more with organophosphates whereas RBC-ChE is associated with nerve agents. After being aged, BChE returns to normal at a rate of approximately 1%/day as the blood cells are replaced. RNC-BChE returns to normal over approximately 50 days. In Tokyo, after the sarin exposure in the subway, a BChE of less than 20% was found to indicate a poor outcome for the patient.

Nerve agents have been used in relatively recent years. As previously noted, in 1994, a cult in Japan called Aum Shinrikyo released sarin in a neighborhood in an attempt to murder local judges. Seven died and 280 victims were injured. One year later, the cult again released and diluted sarin in the Tokyo subway system. The agent was placed in lunch boxes. Members left these boxes on the subway during rush hour and poked holes in them with sharpened umbrellas. There were 11 deaths and

WHY IS IT IMPORTANT **To Be Knowledgeable About Nerve Agents?**

Although nerve agents may seem like a remote possibility, this may not be true. They have been used in the wars in the Middle East and in developed countries such as Japan in recent history. In the past, their use may have been limited by the danger they posed to the terrorist; with the increase in suicide attacks, this may not be as great a concern.

5500 injured, both commuters and first responders.[9] It is extremely important to note that 85% of the victims presented directly to the health-care facility without waiting for emergency medical services or decontamination.

Vesicants

Mustards and lewisite are vesicating agents that cause burns and blisters, a very simplistic way of looking at these agents; they have far more devastating systemic effects. Mustards are liquids at typical environmental temperatures. They are oily, yellow-brown, and heavier than water. They smell like mustard, (where they get their name), garlic, onions, or horseradish. As gasses, they are heavier than air and will accumulate in low-lying areas; they may persist in the environment for weeks, depending on conditions.[10,11]

It is speculated that mustards cause cell death and injury in one or more of four possible ways. Mustards appear to cause alkylation of deoxyribonucleic acid (DNA). This causes DNA strands to break, which may cause unbalanced function and the production of proteinase leading to cell death, damage, or blister formation. It also inhibits separation of DNA strands, which inhibits replication necessary for cell division. In this way, mustards have a greater effect on rapidly growing cells. Mustards also create oxidative stress on cells either through depletion of glutathione that normally detoxifies reactive oxygen species or through diffusion across cellular membranes causing a calcium imbalance, loss of cellular integrity, and cellular death. This is most present in moist environments such as the lungs and eyes. Finally, mustards produce a significant inflammatory response.[11]

Signs and Symptoms

Mustards have a potentially devastating effect on their victims; however, effects may not be immediate and may be delayed for hours or longer. Because of this, the victims or rescuers may not feel a sense of urgency and immediately seek decontamination. Mustards affect the skin approximately 2 to 4 hours after exposure. Those areas prone to sweating such as the groin and axilla will be affected first followed by other exposed areas, including the eyes and respiratory tract. Mustards are highly soluble in fat so they travel easily along sweat glands and hair follicles and affect the upper respiratory tract. Skin effects are directly related to the area exposed, even under clothing and the amount of exposure to the agent. The amount of exposure to the agent is related to the ambient temperature. As with nerve agents, warmer temperatures cause more of the agent to be off-gassed leading to higher concentrations in the air. Initial reaction is erythema approximately 2 to 4 hours after exposure. Severe pruritus is present at this time, but resolves as blisters form in about 18 to 24 hours. Mustards affect the endothelium of capillaries and venules causing leakage of vascular fluid. The agent then affects the DNA of the epidermal layer of the skin further causing vascular leakage, neutrophilic immigration, and ulceration. The effects on the skin should be characterized as similar to thermal burns except the burns from mustard take at least twice as long to heal.[10,11]

The eyes become inflamed several hours after exposure. Mustards are readily absorbed by the conjunctiva and cornea. Victims develop spasmodic blinking (blepharospasm), eye pain, tearing, photophobia, and blurred vision. There will be periorbital edema and conjunctival injection. Injuries may be considered as mild, moderate, or severe. Mild injuries will have little corneal involvement with mild erythema and conjunctivitis. There will be irritation but little tearing. The victim should recover in several days. Moderate eye injury involves the cornea, conjunctiva, and eye lids. Symptoms of dry eyes, photophobia, pain, and possibly blindness occur approximately 6 hours after exposure. There will be periorbital edema, the eye lids may swell together, and there will be spasmodic blinking. Some of the symptoms will lessen over 48 hours; however, it may take as long as 6 weeks for full recovery. Severe injuries involve full thickness corneal burns, severe pain, spamming, and blurred vision. The cornea will have an orange peel effect and may lack sensitivity; other injuries may occur including necrosis. There may not be resolution for 1 to 2 weeks for the symptoms with other effects lasting up to 40 years.[10,11]

The effect of mustards on the respiratory system is the most common cause of death and is an extreme source of discomfort for the victims who survive. Mild exposures cause chest tightness and cough. Moderate-to-severe exposures cause sneezing, nasal discharge and bleeding, sore throat, hoarseness, and a hacking cough that may last for 10 to 48 hours. The cough may or may not produce sputum. Pulmonary edema and bronchial pneumonia then appears. Bronchial and tracheal pseudomembranes develop and begin to slough off, further blocking the airway. Long-term effects include the development of reactive airway disease, pulmonary fibrosis, interstitial lung disease, emphysema, and airway obstruction.[10,11]

Lewisite

Lewisite is a colorless odorless liquid; impurities may make it amber or a brownish color. It is heavier than mustard and does not mix well with water. Lewisite is both a vesicant and systemic poison. Its vesicant effects occur much faster than those of mustard. At levels as low as 8 mg/min/m^3, the victim may experience irritation of the respiratory tract. This is significantly lower than the level required to detect its odor, that of geraniums at a level of 20 mg/min/m^3. Lewisite is readily absorbed through the skin and as little as 2 mL can be fatal to an adult. As a systemic poison it affects the liver, gallbladder, kidneys, and urinary tract. It has a high affinity for several enzymes and affects vascular permeability leading to volume loss and shock.[10,11]

Signs and Symptoms

Table 9–4 compares phosgene and lewisite. Lewisite affects the skin within 10 to 20 seconds causing discomfort. The discomfort progresses to a deep aching pain. Erythema occurs within 15 to 30 minutes and vesication in about 12 to 18 hours. These burns are significantly deeper and more difficult to heal than those of mustards. Eye pain is significant and eyes may swell shut within an hour. Corneal damage may occur, particularly at higher doses. Airways may experience a burning sensation followed by significant increase in secretions. Productive cough, epistaxis, frothy mucus, laryngitis, and dyspnea also are common. As with mustard, pseudomembranes may develop, leading to airway obstruction. Gastrointestinal symptoms include nausea and vomiting from either inhalation or ingestion. Hepatic necrosis and renal failure may occur. As stated, hypovolemic shock may occur related to increased vascular permeability and subsequent fluid loss.[10,11]

Treatment of Lewisite and Mustards

If the agent is known, Level B or C protective equipment should be worn for the decontamination process. If the agent is unknown, Level A protective equipment should be used. After decontamination has been completed, standard precautions include Class D protective equipment and standard universal precautions.

TABLE 9–4 The Difference and Similarities of Phosgene and Lewisite

MUSTARDS	LEWISITE
Affects the skin in 2 to 4 hours.	Affects skin in 10 to 29 seconds.
Erythema in 2 to 4 hours.	Erythema in 15 to 30 minutes.
Vesication in 18 to 24 hours.	Vesication in 12 to 18 hours.
Eyes significant spasmodic blinking, swelling, and discomfort after several hours.	Eyes significant swelling in 1 hour with significant pain.
Chest tightness and cough, sneezing, nasal discharge and bleeding, sore throat, hoarseness and a hacking cough that may last for 10 to 48 hours. Cough may or may not produce sputum. Pulmonary edema and bronchial pneumonia then appear. Bronchial and tracheal pseudomembranes develop and begin to slough off further blocking the airway.	Productive cough, epistaxis, frothy mucus, laryngitis, and dyspnea. Bronchial and tracheal pseudomembranes develop and begin to slough off further blocking the airway.

In contrast to those affected by mustards, victims of lewisite experience discomfort shortly after exposure so they are more likely to seek decontamination quickly. For both agents, it is important to decontaminate eyes and skin as quickly as possible. Eyes should be flushed for 5 to 10 minutes and skin washed with soap and water. It also may be necessary to use hypochlorite acid (bleach), flour, or talc on skin. British anti-lewisite (BAL) is the antidote specific to lewisite. It acts as a chelating agent but has significant side effects of its own. It should be used only in those patients exhibiting shock or significant pulmonary injury. Supportive care is essential for victims including oxygen, possible intubation, and bronchoscopy to clear the airway. Burns are very difficult to heal and will take much longer than thermal burns. Debridement of the burns and application of Silvadene cream are both appropriate.[10,11]

Off-gassing from clothing or skin of the victim may occur. This places rescue and treating personnel at risk. Anyone coming in contact with a victim of lewisite should use Level A protection including self-contained breathing apparatus.

Class II Agents

Class II agents are those agents that have significant use in industry, but may also be used as weapons. Three of these agents are cyanide, chlorine, and phosgene.

Cyanide

Cyanide is used extensively in industry. Chemical synthesis, electroplating, metallurgy, printing, tanning, agriculture, photography, paper, plastics, and insecticides are a few industrial applications in which various forms of cyanide are used. For terrorist considerations, both the volatility of some of the forms and the availability of the agent or its waste products make it very attractive. Besides terrorist threats, responders and health-care personnel should be concerned about potential spills and smoke inhalation from fires. Hydrogen cyanide (HCN) may be produced from the combustion of many synthetic plastics. Any material that contains carbon and nitrogen can produce cyanide when burned. Victims of smoke and carbon dioxide exposure also may be victims of cyanide poisoning.[10,12]

Cyanide as a poison has been used since ancient times. It was first isolated in 1782. Napoleon III coated bayonets with cyanide for battle during the Franco-Prussian war. It was used ineffectively in World War I. In World War II, it was used by the Nazis in the death camps. It is widely available in many formulas and forms, which may increase its potential as a chemical weapon; it certainly increases the potential for accidental release.

HCN is extremely volatile and readily evaporates into a gaseous state. It is lighter than air so outside of a contained area it would disperse easily. This makes it a poor candidate for terrorist activities in other than an enclosed environment. In an enclosed area, the high volatility would make it a significant threat. Cyanogen chloride was developed specifically to overcome the shortcomings of HCN for use as a weapon. It is heavier than air and less volatile; this makes it more persistent, slow to dissipate, and more significant as a weapon.[10,12]

Signs and Symptoms

The time it takes for symptoms to occur, the severity of the symptoms, and how lethal the incident is depends on both the type of cyanide and its form. Gaseous inhalation produces the most rapid onset with ingestion being the most delayed. An exception to this is mercurial cyanide salts. The mercurial component is extremely toxic and will have immediate affects if ingested.

Cyanide is normally found in our environment; it is present in small amounts in cigarette smoke and some foods. Our bodies are generally well equipped to metabolize this small amount of cyanide exposure; we are not equipped to metabolize large amounts and are quickly overwhelmed. Cyanide binds with Fe^{3+} at the mitochondrial level and prevents the transport and utilization of oxygen. This leads to anaerobic energy production and the buildup of lactic acid. Cyanide crosses the blood-brain barrier easily and after across may interfere with neurotransmitters. It also increases intravascular resistance. Early signs of cyanide poisoning may be evident in as little as a few minutes.

Early signs and symptoms include dizziness, headache, weakness, diaphoresis, and rapid respirations. There will be a transient increase in blood pressure. It is important to note that these signs and symptoms are not very specific and may be confused with the presentation of other complaints such as anxiety. The victim may state that they detected an odor of bitter almonds or they may have a cherry red flush. These may or may not be present in all cases. Because the effect of cyanide poisoning is to block the use of oxygen at the cellular level, venous blood oxygen levels will approach that of arterial blood. Ophthalmic examination will reveal that both retinal arteries and veins will appear the same.[10,12]

Arterial and venous blood gasses will equalize in oxygen content. As hypoxia continues, victims will exhibit decreasing level of consciousness progressing to unresponsiveness. They will progress through hemodynamic instability, arrhythmias, seizures, apnea, and cardiac arrest. Throughout all of this, the oxygen saturation of the blood will remain high. Chronic exposure may produce ataxia, anoxic encephalopathy, dystonia, and Parkinson-like symptoms. Testing of the environment or the patient is difficult and the results may be delayed or inaccurate. Treatment should be based on presentation and index of suspicion.

Evidence for Practice

Treatment of victims of cyanide poisoning should be based on presentation and index of suspicion. Victims will exhibit progressive signs of hypoxia in spite of normal arterial oxygen saturation. Venous oxygen levels will equalize with arterial because cyanide prevents oxygen utilization at the cellular level.

Treatment

If the agent is known, Level B or C protective equipment should be worn for the decontamination process. If the agent is unknown, Level A protective equipment should be used. Personnel should wear at least level C personal protective equipment during treatment to avoid becoming affected by residual cyanide present on the victim's clothing and skin as well as through the victim's breathing.

Treatment includes immediate decontamination. Remove the victim from the toxin; this is particularly important for gaseous forms of cyanide. Remove the victim's clothing and jewelry and place these in a plastic bag with the victim's name or identification number on it. Tap water, normal saline, or lactated Ringer's may be used to flush the victim's eyes. If ingestion has occurred, do not induce vomiting because this has shown to increase mortality. If the ingestion occurred less than 1 hour earlier, the victim may be given activated charcoal. One gram of charcoal absorbs approximately 35 mg of cyanide. This may be enough to save the victim's life.[10]

Medical treatment begins with supporting the victim's breathing and hemodynamic function. Placing the victim on oxygen is important. They may not be able to completely utilize the supplemental oxygen because of the effects of cyanide at the cellular level, but any mitochondria not affected should be given the opportunity to use the oxygen as efficiently as possible. Although there is some evidence to support placing the victim in hyperbaric oxygen, this remains controversial. Lactic acid will begin to build up from anaerobic metabolism and should be treated. The victim will develop seizures, which may be extremely difficult to treat.[10]

Medications in the United States used to treat cyanide poisoning include amyl nitrite, sodium nitrite, and sodium thiosulfate. Amyl nitrite is supplied as an ampule that is broken into a gauze pad and inhaled. It is placed under the victim's nose for 30 seconds out of each 60 seconds. Replace the ampule every 3 minutes. Sodium nitrite is given as 10 cc (300 mg) over 5 minutes. These medications are given to create a state of methemoglobinemia. Cyanide binds preferably to methemoglobin, which leaves the mitochondria to function normally. Side effects of these medications include hypotension due to vasodilatation. This may exacerbate the effect of cardiovascular medications the victim may already be on. Sodium thiosulfate binds reversibly to cyanide facilitating its clearing. Side effects are rare but include hypersensitivity or hypotension. Hydroxycobalamin is given as a 5-g IV dose. It reacts with cyanide to form cyanocobalamin, vitamin B_{12}, and is eliminated from the body. Side effects include transient flushing and hypertension.[10,12]

Chlorine and Phosgene

Chlorine and phosgene are toxic gasses that are widely used and available both in industry and municipal settings. Phosgene is used in the manufacturing of dyes, pesticides, plastics, polyurethane, and pharmaceuticals. It also is identified by several names including carbonyl chloride, carbon oxychloride, oxychloride, and carbonic acid chloride. CG is the military designation for phosgene.

Chlorine is used extensively in cleaning, disinfection, and the manufacturing of synthetics and plastics. Chlorine is most often the chemical accidentally released in both industry and household settings. The ease of obtaining chlorine and the fact that both chlorine and phosgene are transported and stored in large quantities make both attractive to terrorist groups. Beyond terrorist potential, these agents have a very high potential for devastating accidents.[11]

Chlorine is gaseous at –34°C (–29°F) and phosgene is a gas at 8°C (47°F). Chlorine is gaseous at environmental temperatures but is stored under pressure as a liquid. Phosgene may be encountered as either a liquid or a gas; both are a concern. The amount of these agents in the environment after a release is dependent on air movement and humidity. Both agents would be dispersed by a strong wind; however, both are heavier than air and would collect in low-lying areas. Chlorine causes airway irritation at 30 parts per million (ppm). Slightly higher concentrations, 40 ppm for 30 minutes may cause severe lung injury.[11] Exposures of 500 ppm for 5 minutes may cause lethal injury. Chlorine is an irritant and requires significant exposure time at low concentrations to be lethal whereas phosgene's level of toxic exposure occurs before it is noticed. Phosgene produces the odor of new mown hay at 0.4 ppm. Exposure below this level for a significant amount of time may be toxic. LCt 50 for phosgene is 500 to 800 ppm for 2 minutes.[11]

Signs and Symptoms

Chlorine is very soluble in water, forming hydrochloric and hypochlorous acids. It reacts early in the airway and causes most of its damage there. Other moist areas such as the eyes are affected. Phosgene does not react as easily with water and exhibits its effects within the lower respiratory tract where it often reacts as small amount of hydrogen chloride and hydroxyl groups through acylation. These hydroxyl groups disrupt cellular membranes and enzyme function. Chlorine also disrupts the surfactant layer impairing lung function. Inflammation occurs. If the concentration is high enough, greater than 500 ppm, the effects become systemic causing hemolysis and red blood cell hyperaggregation. Pulmonary sludging occurs leading to cor pulmonale and death.[11]

Primary effects of both of these agents is to the respiratory system causing airway obstruction, interstitial damage, and alveolar/capillary damage, and impairing gas exchange. High enough concentrations may displace enough environmental oxygen to cause asphyxiation. Chlorine is highly irritating and will cause coughing and pain in eyes and throat. Because of this, victims will attempt to leave the area quickly. Victims also will develop headache, excessive salivation, dyspnea, hemoptysis, burning in the chest, and vomiting. Symptoms lessen with time. Treatment includes protecting the airway

Evidence for Practice

Victims of chlorine gas exposure will seek to remove themselves from the area quickly because of the irritating effects of the gas; victims of phosgene may be exposed to lethal doses and not be aware. The scent of new mown hay (phosgene) appears at higher concentrations than those required for a lethal exposure.

and examination via bronchoscopy. Practitioners should be prepared to provide an emergency airway.[11]

Phosgene has a more insidious effect **(see Table 9–5)**. As stated there may initially be only a mild cough. Examination of records from World War I indicate that the shorter the latency period the more significant the injury. This latent period may range from 2 to 15 hours. Pulmonary edema and decreased oxygen saturation may lag behind the patients with dyspnea. Rapid progressive and possibly profound pulmonary edema may occur leading to hypotension and rapid significant volume loss from alveolar capillaries. Fluid management for these patients is difficult but essential for recovery. The development of pulmonary edema in the first 2 to 4 hours is indicative of poor prognosis.[11]

Treatment

If the agent is known, Level B or C protective equipment should be worn for the decontamination process. If the agent is unknown, Level A protective equipment should be used. After decontamination has been completed use standard precautions that include Level D protective equipment and standard universal precautions.

TABLE 9–5 Chlorine and Phosgene Effects and Treatment	
CHLORINE	PHOSGENE
Airway irritant.	Odor of new mown hay.
Immediate effects at low concentrations.	Lethal dose possible before victims are aware.
Forms hypochlorous acid causing bronchospasm, hemolysis, pulmonary sludge, RBC aggregation, cor pulmonale, and death.	Begins with a mild cough, latent period of 2 to 15 hours, followed by rapid progressive pulmonary edema, significant fluid loss.
Airway control, inhaled beta-agonist inhalers controlling bronchospasm.	Hemodynamic monitoring and fluid management, beta-agonist inhalers, limited use of diuretics.

Treatment for exposure to both of these agents is supportive with a few important caveats. Airway control is of primary concern. Particularly with chlorine, injury and the development of bronchospasm is progressive. Patients should be monitored closely both before and after presentation to the hospital. Treatment may include salbutamol and beta agonist inhalers; however, particularly in the case of phosgene, a normal oxygen saturation may not indicate positive prognosis. For chlorine, a nebulized solution of 3.5% to 5% sodium bicarbonate may be helpful. There also may be transient cardiac arrhythmias but they should be limited and resolve with oxygenation. Treatment of pulmonary edema should mimic that of adult respiratory distress syndrome (ARDS). The use of diuretics will have limited positive effect and will only contribute to volume depletion. Patients may lose up to 1 liter of fluid per hour to capillary leakage. Fluid resuscitation and positive-pressure ventilation with positive end-expiratory pressure (PEEP) and inhaled or systemic steroids are required to support oxygenation and treatment of the progressive pulmonary edema.[11]

Laboratory tests and chest x-rays (CXRs) are of little initial value. Arterial blood gases (ABGs) upon presentation will be relatively normal. They may only indicate an elevated P_{CO_2}, which would be expected of a patient with reactive airway. The normal oxygen level will be falsely reassuring, particularly in the case of phosgene. CXR may be useful only as a baseline for further studies. It may be helpful a few hours after exposure to assist with the diagnosis of pulmonary edema. Chlorine exposure may produce atelectasis relayed to its effects on upper airways and phosgene may produce hyperinflation from its effects on lower, smaller airways. Moderate-to-high exposures to phosgene may produce radiological findings in 1 to 2 hours. Early findings are indicative of much sicker victims. A CXR that remains clear for 8 hours usually indicates that the victim will not develop pulmonary edema.[11]

In subsequent days, patients may develop elevated white blood cell counts and infiltrates on CXR. Although this may be indicative of an opportunistic infection, it may not have a bacterial cause. Sputum cultures may be helpful to guide treatment. Treatment may also be guided by the progression of these markers. If the infiltrates worsen over 3 or more days, they may be indicative of a bacterial or viral infection and should be treated appropriately.[11]

An extremely important consideration for phosgene is physical activity. It was found in World War I that physical activity after exposure greatly affects the patient's condition and prognosis. Patients who are quite stable laying flat may worsen significantly when sitting or walking. Any activity that increases oxygen demands on the body, even activity as simple as bathing the patient, may increase lung injury and cause the patient to deteriorate even after they have been asymptomatic.

There are other treatments being investigated but supportive care remains the norm. Symptoms may last for 1 to 9 weeks (in the case of chlorine). Chronic effects, particularly with airway obstructions, are common. Patients who have suffered phosgene exposure may complain of dyspnea and decreased activity tolerance. It may take years to fully recover from exposure.[11]

If the agent is known, Level B or C protective equipment should be worn for the decontamination process. If the agent is unknown, Level A protective equipment should be used. After decontamination has been completed, use standard precautions including Level D protective equipment and standard universal precautions. There is little chance of contamination from victims after they have been removed from the scene.

Class III Agents

There are perhaps hundreds of thousands of Class III agents. They are gases, solids, and liquids used in industrial, medical, and other institutional settings; many can be commonly found

Evidence for Practice

Victims recovering from exposure to phosgene should be allowed very limited physical activity. Any activity that places stress on the body's systems including sitting, walking, and even bathing or being bathed, may worsen the victim's condition significantly.

in households with everyday uses. Bulk transport of cleaning products; oxygen; other gases; fuels; industrial chemicals such as corrosives, flammable or explosive gases and liquids; and poisonous chemicals are carried across the nation by the railroad and trucking industries. Large quantities are stored in institutional and industrial settings. Although spills are relatively rare, the potential exists for accidental or intentional releases that may pose risks for people and the environment. Examining even the most common of these agents is far beyond the scope of this book. There are some guidelines that may be helpful in dealing with spills and releases:

- Unknown agents should be treated with the highest degree of caution until the agent is identified. Subsequent precautions are then based on the toxic agent. Often the agent can be identified through placards on railcars or trucks and supportive documentation. Material Safety Data Sheets (MSDS) are required to be on file wherever toxic agents are being used. These and the supporting literature will identify the agent and specify cleanup and treatment.

- If decontamination is necessary, victims of exposures to Class III agents, as with other agents, should be decontaminated at the scene. Specific methods of decontamination depend on the toxic agent and should be noted in the MSDS sheets. The level of personal protection equipment also will vary depending on the agent.

- Injuries from these agents also vary extensively. Burns, respiratory difficulties, neurological concerns, eye irritation or blindness, and other injuries are common if care is not taken to immediately contain spills and evacuate the area. Nursing and health-care providers must be aware of common chemicals stored, used or transported in the area where they practice and their effects.

Summary

The possibility of intentional or accidental release of chemical agents and the potential harm from the release ranges from slight to significant. Areas near industrial centers or major transportation hubs and infrastructure may be at high risk for various potential releases. Other areas may be at relatively low risk from a few well-defined chemicals used locally. Any part of the country or world is at risk for intentional release of a wide variety of agents that can be devastating. Performing a risk assessment to identify common chemicals used, stored, or transported through an area is extremely important in disaster planning for industry, health care, and the community as a whole. If a particular agent is used extensively in local industry or regularly transported through the area, specific protocols should be established by industry, health-care facilities, and the community for care of victims and cleanup. These protocols include the following:

- Identifying the level of protective equipment that should be used.
- Creating evacuation areas and plans.
- Estimating numbers of potential victims and the protocols necessary to treat them.
- Identifying specific treatments and the supplies needed to care for the victims.
- Preparing clean-up procedures to minimize the environmental impact.

These protocols will allow community leaders and health-care providers—EMS, physicians, nurse practitioners, nurses, and other personnel—to work quickly and effectively in controlling a toxic spill and treating its victims.

Nursing administration and practitioners in the emergency department should work with local industry, EMS, and the emergency department to prepare these protocols. This would provide prompt treatment beginning at the scene of the incident and carrying through presentation to the emergency department and possible hospital admission. In the end, preparation for possible spills is essential for prompt response and effective treatment.

1. Kenar L, Karayilanoglu T. Prehospital management and medical intervention after a chemical attack. *Emergency Medicine Journal.* 2004;21(1):84–88.

2. Powers R. Organization of a hospital-based victim decontamination plan using the incident command structure. *Disaster Management and Response: DMR.* 2007;5(4):19–123.

3. Severance HW. Mass-casualty victim "surge" management. Preparing for bombings and blast-related injuries with possibility of hazardous materials exposure. *North Carolina Medical Journal.* 2002;63(5):242–246.

4. Karayilanoglu T, Kenar L, Gulec M. Evaluations over the medical emergency responding to chemical terrorist attack. *Military Medicine.* 2003;168(8):591–594.

5. Koenig KL, Boatright CJ, Hancock JA, et al. Health care facility-based decontamination of victims exposed to chemical, biological, and radiological materials. *American Journal of Emergency Medicine.* 2008;26(1):71–80.

6. Ben Abraham R, Weinbroum AA. Resuscitative challenges in nerve agent poisoning. *European Journal of Emergency Medicine.* 2003;10(3):169–175.

7. Barelli A, Biondi I, Soave M, Tafani C, Bononi F. The comprehensive medical preparedness in chemical emergencies: 'the chain of chemical survival'. *European Journal of Emergency Medicine.* 2008;15(2):110–118.

8. Levitin HW, Siegelson HJ, Dickinson S, et al. Decontamination of mass casualties—re-evaluating existing dogma. *Prehospital and Disaster Medicine.* 2003;18(3):200–207.

9. Veenema TG, ed. *Disaster Nursing and Emergency Preparedness for Chemical, Biological and Radiological Terrorism and Other Hazards.* 2nd ed. New York, NY: Springer; 2007.

10. Noeller TP. Biological and chemical terrorism: recognition and management. *Cleveland Clinic Journal of Medicine.* 2004;68(12):1001–1002.

11. Muskat PC. Mass casualty chemical exposure and implications for respiratory failure. *Respiratory Care.* 2008;53(1):58–63; discussion 63–66.

12. Keim ME. Terrorism involving cyanide: the prospect of improving preparedness in the prehospital setting. *Prehospital and Disaster Medicine.* 2006;21(2 Suppl 2):S56–S60.

Weapons of Mass Destruction Explosives

10

Introduction

Arguably the most-used weapon of terrorism throughout the world is explosives. One of the most potent weapons of mass destruction (WMD) is nuclear weapons. Improvised explosive devices (IEDs) are used extensively in the Iraq and Afghanistan wars and have become very sophisticated. Suicide bombers, now including women and teenagers, cause significant destruction worldwide. To date, the most significant attacks in the United States, London, and Spain have involved explosives. As weapons of terror, they are relatively easy to obtain, make, and use. They are particularly easy to deploy effectively when used by suicide terrorists **(see Fig. 10–1).**

Nursing and medicine in the military deal with traumatic injuries from the initial trauma to the potentially long recovery on a daily basis; this is not the case for most health-care providers in civilian life. Although the health-care system certainly deals with trauma related to motor vehicle accidents, transportation and industrial accidents, and other traumas, it does not often deal with the unique injuries associated with explosives. Nor does it have a good understanding of how explosives work and their potential to do harm. It is very important that nursing education teach a basic understanding of explosives and the injuries associated with them and relate this information to basic nursing course work concerning patient care. It is also important that nurses practicing as registered nurses and as advanced practice nurses continue to expand this basic understanding as it applies to their practice. This includes emergency care, intensive care, medical and surgical care, recovery, and rehabilitation. Nursing administration should provide support for these activities and encourage education both in formal educational programs and continuing education programs throughout practice. Explosive trauma like many illness and traumas mentioned in this book are relatively rare; however, the skills used to provide care for victims are used relatively frequently. Nursing and the medical community need an understanding of what may occur and why, the preparations required for potentially large numbers of victims, and how to apply this knowledge to practice.

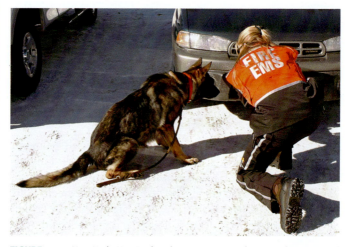

FIGURE 10–1. New York, New York, February 12, 2002. The Westminster Kennel Club honored the canine heroes of 9-11 during the club's 126th Dog Show in a ceremony at Madison Square Garden. But the work of these canines goes on. Nikko, a trained explosives detection dog, works with Shawn Winder of the Park City Fire District on a mock explosives exercise in Solitude, Utah, at the Winter Olympics. Explosives are the most common terrorist weapon, bomb sniffing dogs are one tool in the fight against terrorism. *Photo by Andrea Booher/FEMA News Photo.*

ALERT!

Explosives are the most common weapon used by terrorists. They are extremely easy to deploy and can cause extensive damage. With the increase in suicide bombers, which now include women and children, this threat becomes even more significant. Secondary explosions after the primary explosion are intended to cause injury to those responding to care for the victims of the first explosion. Health-care providers must be aware of the types of injuries and the extent of the danger created by the use of explosives.

Types of Explosives

This section covers types of explosives. Explosives can be classified into conventional and nuclear explosives. There are some similarities but nuclear explosives are significantly more destructive than conventional explosives. Conventional explosives depend on a chemical reaction that turns solids or liquids into energy extremely quickly and releases heat and creates pressure waves. Conventional explosives are further classified as low-power, high-power, and incendiary devices. Nuclear weapons depend on a reaction at the atomic level. The atom of the nuclear material is split apart, nuclear fission, or forced together, as in nuclear fusion. In both cases, a new element is created and tremendous amounts of heat, pressure, and radioactive material are expelled. A variation that uses a conventional explosive to spread radioactive material over an area is called a dirty bomb.

Conventional

Conventional explosives can be classified in multiple ways; low-power explosives such as gun powder can be differentiated from high-explosives such as plastic explosives/SEMTEX. Explosives also can be differentiated from incendiary devices.[1–3]

Low and high explosives differ in how quickly the explosive material is converted into energy. Low explosives burn quickly releasing gas and heat. Their explosive nature results from confining this energy within a shell that then ruptures or explodes. The process is referred to as deflagration and can occur quite rapidly. Low explosives are often used as propellants or in pyrotechnics and flares.[1–3]

Low explosives deflagrate at rates of about 400 meters/second and high explosives convert to energy at rates of 4000 meters/second. The conversion of material into gas and heat takes place in a millisecond effectively causing the material itself to detonate. High explosives are rated according to their brisance. Brisance refers to the shattering or breaking power of the explosive. Low explosives may cause the ripping apart of their containers; however, high explosives would shatter or pulverize the container. The measure of how quickly an explosive reaches its peak pressure is its brisance. This rapid conversion of matter into energy and incredibly expanding sphere of gas creates an overpressure wave or blast wave, and a dynamic wave; further differentiating it from low explosives[1–3] **(see Fig. 10–2).**

Incendiary devices differ from explosive devices in that they are meant to burn, possibly at extremely high temperatures. The devices range from the very simple such as Molotov cocktails to armor piercing weapons that ignite after piercing armor plating. Molotov cocktails are made of gasoline or other volatile liquid contained in a glass bottle with a fuse, usually a piece of cloth attached to the opening. Once the fuse is lit, the bottle is thrown, shatters and causes the contents to ignite. Metals such as iron, aluminum, or magnesium also may be used in incendiary devices. While these metals are difficult to ignite as a solid piece, as filings or shavings, they can be ignited relatively easily and burn at extremely high temperatures. Magnesium burns at 2200°C or 4000°F and may use nitrogen or carbon dioxide instead of oxygen as it burns. Incendiaries used during World War II caused significant terror and destruction. Other examples of incendiaries include white phosphorus, napalm (used extensively in World War II, the Korean conflict, and from aerial assaults in the Vietnam War), and kerosene-fueled weapons.[3]

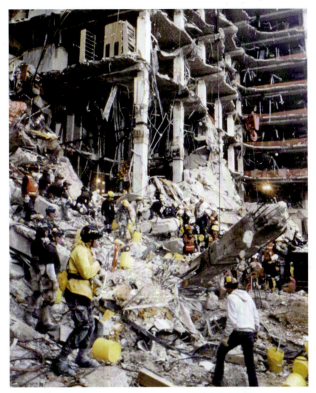

FIGURE 10–2. Oklahoma City, Oklahoma, April 26, 1995. High-powered explosives can cause devastating damage. Here search and rescue crews work to save those trapped beneath the debris, following the Oklahoma City bombing. *FEMA News Photo.*

Nuclear Weapons

Nuclear explosives can be classified as either fission or fusion devices. Fission devices were the first to be developed. They require an unstable isotope such as uranium-235 or plutonium to be of a critical mass and configured to sustain a nuclear reaction. They are triggered by one of two methods. The "gun method" shoots a piece of subcritical fissile material, uranium-235 or plutonium, into another subcritical piece, creating a critical mass and causing sustained nuclear fission.

TABLE 10–1   Types of Explosives

Conventional	Low power	Deflagrate or burn at speeds of 400 m/sec. Used in fireworks and as propellants.
	High power	Stable explosives that convert to heat and gas instantaneously, 4000 m/sec. Measured in brisance or shattering power.
	Incendiary	Burns at temperatures reaching 2200°C. May be able to use nitrogen or carbon dioxide as fuel instead of oxygen.
Nuclear	Fission	The splitting of an atom by striking it with a neutron. Temperatures reaching tens of millions of degrees.
	Fusion	The fusing of atoms into a new element. Initiated by a fission device. Theoretically no limit to the yield or strength of a fusion device.
Dirty Bombs		Conventional explosives packed with radioactive material meant to contaminate the surrounding area.

The implosion method uses chemical explosives to compress a fossil of uranium-235 or plutonium into critical mass[4] **(see Fig. 10–3).**

Fusion devices use a fission device to create the heat and pressure that cause the fusion to occur. These devices may be staged devices. First a fission explosion compresses and heats the fusion material setting off the fusion reaction through the release of gamma and x-rays. The fusion reaction then releases enormous numbers of high-speed neutrons that in turn cause fission of material not prone to fission, such as depleted uranium. Fusion material cannot be made supercritical no matter how much is used and depleted uranium is also subcritical; therefore, a large amount of material can be used thereby

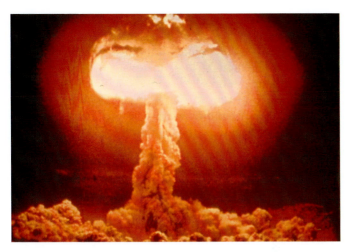

FIGURE 10–3. Nuclear explosions release a tremendous amount of energy in the form of heat and radioactivity in addition to the force of the blast wave. Devastation is widespread, radioactive fallout affects not only those immediately downwind from the explosion but may be carried to other countries by prevailing winds in the upper atmosphere. *FEMA News Photo.*

increasing the yield of fusion weapons significantly beyond that of fission weapons. The yield of fission weapons may range up to 500,000 tons (500 kilotons) of trinitrotoluene (TNT). The largest fusion weapon exploded had a yield of 50 million tons (50 megatons) of TNT.[4]

Two other weapons are worth mentioning as variations in this category. Neutron bombs are designed to have a relatively small explosive yield but significant amounts of neutron radiation. This will cause destruction of the population but leave the infrastructure intact. Nuclear weapons also may be seeded with gold or cobalt, which then produces large quantities of radioactive contamination.[1]

Dirty Bombs

Dirty bombs are conventional explosives that use the explosion to disperse radioactive material. It is not a nuclear explosion. Dirty bombs contaminate the surrounding area with whatever radioactive material is packed around the explosives. The nuclear material most accessible is low-level nuclear waste. It is speculated that this is the material that would be used in a dirty bomb explosion. External radioactive contaminate is easily removed through decontamination. Simple brushing away of loose material and removal of the victims clothing removes 80% to 90% of the contamination. Inhalation or ingestion of the dust may cause more harm: however, the most significant injuries caused by a dirty bomb would be those caused by the blast itself.[1-4]

Blast Physics

When high explosives explode, all of the material is instantaneously converted from an unstable compound to a more stable one, usually a gas. A byproduct of this is the release of energy, usually in the form of heat. As the gas and heat expand, they compress the air surrounding the explosion and form an ever-expanding shock wave. This shock wave has a few very important characteristics. It travels initially at supersonic speeds but slows rapidly and creates an overpressure that also peaks near the explosion and lessens significantly as it speeds out from the explosion. This blast or shock wave has two components: one, the short burst of high but decreasing positive overpressure and two, a negative under-pressure phase that is up to ten-times longer but of a much lower pressure

---

ALERT!

Dirty bombs kill and injure most of their victims through the force of the explosion. They do not make people or structures around them radioactive. After the contamination is removed, the victim and surrounding area are no longer contaminated and poses no threat through radiation. It is thought that low-level radioactive material would be the most likely material used in a dirty bomb because it is most common.

Possibly the most significant effect of a dirty bomb would be the panic it would cause. Victims who are contaminated, those who believe they are contaminated, even those seriously injured from the blast will mistakenly believe they need to be decontaminated immediately in order to survive. In all cases, decontamination should wait until life-threatening injuries of the victim are stabilized.

differential.[1–3,5–10] These are followed by cycles of positive and negative waves of significantly less magnitude.[3]

The actions of both the positive-pressure and negative-pressure phases cause a blast wind to form, first moving outward from the explosion and then back in with the negative phase. This blast wind is formed in two ways. First, the energy of the blast wave compresses and propels the air molecules outward from the blast and second; the area of high pressure formed by the wave of overpressure causes the air to move, as it would from any area of high pressure, to an area of low pressure. The wind reverses direction quickly and rushes back into the blast area to fill the vacuum left by the blast. Depending on the size of the blast this wind can cycle through both phases in a split second or last seconds in each and may reach speeds of 100 kph. Lastly, the fireball created by the explosion expands outward. It is an area of quick and very intense heat causing structures and clothing to begin burning. It also diminishes quickly as it moves out from the explosion.[1–3,6–10]

Blast Pressures

The blast wave can be described as having two aspects: the peak overpressure wave and the dynamic pressure wave. The peak overpressure wave is the increase in pressure compared with the ambient pressure at a given distance and time. The blast wave moves at supersonic speeds away from the blast eventually becoming a conventional sound wave.[5–7,9] Initial speeds may range from 3000 to 8000 meters/second. At these speeds, the wave would pass over a football field in under one sixty-fourth to one-sixteenth of a second. This increase in pressure compresses the air molecules as it moves out from the blast creating a blast front. As stated, this decreases dramatically with distance from the blast. The dynamic pressure wave is the effect of the pressure front and air movement out from the blast. It is the blast wind created by the blast. The overpressure wave from 1 kg of TNT would be 100 psi at 1 meter. At 5 meters, it would be 3 psi and at 10 meters, 1.5 psi. The dynamic wave would be significantly less. At 1 meter, 10 psi; 5 meters, 0.15 psi; and 10 meters, 0.012 psi. The waves also may be reflected off any perpendicular object they encounter including walls, buildings, the ground, the inside of vehicles, even body armor. The reflected waves have an additive effect with the initial blast wave creating higher overpressures, winds, and damage. These combined overpressures may be two- to nine-times stronger than the original blast wave[1–3,5–9] **(see Table 10–2).**

A third type of pressure is the static pressure created by the blast. If the blast were to occur in the open, there would be a momentary increase in static pressure around the blast that would quickly dissipate. When a blast occurs in a confined area, the pressure buildup within the confined space creates a sudden significant increase in static pressure. The effect of this increase depends on the structure and the venting of the pressure and blast.[1–3,5,7,9]

A blast in an enclosed space would cause the static pressure to rise and remain high. The overpressure wave would pass out from the blast and reflect back off of walls, ceilings, and the floor. The dynamic wave would also reflect and both waves would build as they combine with the reflected waves. The combination of increased and prolonged static pressures and the increased overpressure and dynamic waves would significantly increase the destructive effects of the blast. Explosions inside buildings and busses are far more deadly than open air blasts.[1–3,5–9,11]

TABLE 10–2	Types of Blast Pressures
Blast Wave	Overpressure wave caused by the sudden expansion of hot gases under great pressure and compressing the air in front of it forming a blast wave.
Static Pressure	Sudden increase in ambient pressure caused by an explosion. Dissipates quickly in the open but may cause significant injury in an enclosed space.
Dynamic Wave	Blast wind caused by the force of the explosion, may reach hurricane strength lasting a split second with conventional explosives or several seconds in the case of a nuclear explosion.

279

Weapons of Mass Destruction Explosives

ALERT!

Explosions in an enclosed area such as a building or bus are far more deadly than those in the open. The overpressure wave will be reflected off the sides and roof of the enclosure creating higher overpressures. The static pressure from the explosion will not dissipate easily and remain high. Thermal effects also will be magnified because they will also not be permitted to dissipate easily. All of this will increase primary, secondary, and tertiary injuries for all of the victims.

TABLE 10–3 Types of Injuries From Explosions

TYPE OF INJURY	TYPE OF EXPLOSION	EFFECT OF EXPLOSION ON PATIENT
Primary	Spallation	The effect of the blast wave as it passes through organs of differing densities and reacts near surfaces and boundaries.
	Implosion	The compression and rapid exploding of air-filled spaces in the body such as the ears and sinuses.
	Inertia	The moving of neighboring organs of differing weights and densities at differing speeds.
Secondary		Injuries caused by fragmentation and shrapnel from the explosion. May be penetrating or blunt trauma.
Tertiary		Injuries caused by throwing the victim into stationary objects by the force of the explosion.
Combined		Injuries from all the above in addition to thermal burns from the explosion.

Water creates significant increases in blast waves. Water is not compressible; therefore, no energy is lost as the over-pressure wave moves outward from the blast. Because of this the overpressure wave is faster and remains strong for a much longer time and distance. It may move at speeds up to 5000 ft/sec. The lethal range of an underwater explosion is about three times that of an open air explosion.[1–3,7,9]

The overpressure wave is affected by its travel through different mediums such as water and air and reflected off hard surfaces, it also is affected and affects the body of living creatures. It compresses air in air-filled areas then allows it to expand instantaneously and as it passes through fluids creates tremendous heaving effects.[2–5] These injuries are called primary blast injuries. The position of the body in relation to the blast will affect the extent of the injuries from the overpressure. Bodies with the long axis oriented perpendicular to the blast wave or turned so that the side is facing the blast are most at risk for injury. If they are near a reflecting surface, they are more at risk. Those least at risk would be those who are oriented end on or parallel to the blast wave and not near any reflective surfaces. If in the water, the person least at risk would be floating on the surface, not treading water, but parallel to the surface. Because of the wave's reflection off the surface tension of the water, most damage from an underwater explosion is near but under the surface of the water. The overpressure wave is then released as a heaving of the surface of the water.[1–3,8,9]

Nuclear Blast

Although some of the physics of a nuclear explosion are basically the same as those of non-nuclear blasts, there are some differences and those points in common are magnified exponentially. There is an overpressure wave that extends outward from the blast followed by a negative pressure wave rushing back toward the blast to fill the vacuum. The dynamic wave rushes outward, reverses direction and rushes back toward the blast. These waves can still be and are reflected off of the ground or significant structures that are not destroyed as the waves move outward. There is a fireball though much more intense and incredibly large.

Other aspects are unique to nuclear blasts. Nuclear explosions occur when an unstable isotope reaches critical mass and the capacity to sustain either fission or fusion of the atomic structure. In fission, a neutron enters the nucleus of the atom causing it to split into another element and release other neutrons. In the case of fusion, enough pressure and heat is applied to atoms causing them to fuse together into a new element. Both release a tremendous amount of energy in the process. With fission, the material must be configured in such a way and have enough mass that the released neutrons from one reaction strike the nucleus of other atoms causing them to split and release neutrons, continuing the reaction; this is called critical mass. With fusion, a fission blast provides the needed heat and pressure to begin a sustained reaction.[1,2,4]

At the center of a nuclear explosion temperatures of several tens of millions of degrees centigrade develop immediately; in contrast, conventional weapons produce temperatures of thousands of degrees. The energy released at the moment of the nuclear explosion vaporizes any material that is not part of or has not gone through fission. This radiation released from the fission process is in the form of x-rays, which are absorbed by the surrounding air causing it to become superheated. This forms the intense fireball seen after an explosion. The fireball expands rapidly; a millisecond after the explosion of a 1-megaton burst the fireball is 150 meters across. It reaches its maximum of 2200 meters in about 10 seconds. The rapid expansion of the fireball compresses the surrounding air, forming the blast wave. The blast wave initially travels through superheated air allowing it to move much faster than normal. It initially lags behind the leading edge of the fireball, eventually catching up, momentarily obscuring the leading edge and finally passing it. For this reason, thermal radiation from a nuclear blast has a pulsed affect; an initial burst, followed by a diminishing burst, followed by a stronger burst.[1,2,4] Nuclear explosions cause tremendous increases in static pressure even in the open and the reflective increases in blast waves is amplified simply off the ground creating the Mach effect. The combined overpressures are two- to nine-times stronger and a vertical blast wall extends out from the blast. The positive and negative phases of the blast wave may last several seconds, not simply a split second. The winds of the dynamic wave may reach hurricane force. Structures weakened by the overpressure wave, may be torn apart by the negative pressure immediately behind the positive overpressure and finally destroyed by the dynamic wave or wind as it moves out from the blast, then followed by significant winds moving back into the blast area.[1,6,7]

Nuclear blasts have three major effects: blast, thermal, and radiation. Approximately 50% of the energy is expressed as the blast, 35% as thermal, and 15% as ionizing radiation. Five percent of the ionizing radiation is released in the first minute of the explosion creating the fireball and 10% is released as residual radiation causing radioactive fallout. For a 1 kiloton explosion, 50% of people exposed would be incapacitated at 600 meters with a 50% fatality rate at 800 meters from ionizing radiation. The blast wave would be lethal to 50% of those exposed at 140 meters and the thermal radiation would cause incapacitating second-degree burns to 50% of those exposed at 369 meters.[1,2,4]

Nuclear weapons are exploded either as airbursts, surface bursts, subsurface bursts, or high-altitude bursts. Each has significantly different effects. **High-altitude bursts** cause an intense electromagnetic pulse (EMP). This has a tremendous effect on complex electronic equipment, but has no direct biological effect. There would be no fallout and both the thermal and blast effects would be minimized depending on the height of the blast. **Airburst** explosions are those that occur 30 kilometers above the ground or at a height from which the fireball does not touch the ground. These bursts are maximized for thermal and blast effects, creating the Mach effect of a significantly increased blast wave. Other than radiation effects at ground zero, there is only a slight chance of local radioactive fallout. Most radioactive material is carried globally. **Surface detonations** cause cratering and tremendous destruction at ground zero but significantly less widespread effects than airbursts. Because the fireball touches the surface, large amounts of dirt or water are vaporized, sucked up into the atmosphere and cause significant local radioactive fallout. **Subsurface detonations** will cause cratering and radioactive fallout if the blast breaks the surface, otherwise their effects would be limited to ground shock waves[1,2,4] **(see Fig. 10–4).**

Fallout is a significant effect of nuclear explosions. It takes two forms, local and worldwide fallout. When a nuclear explosion occurs, weapon residuals, unfissionable material and remaining fissionable materials are vaporized. They condense into very small particles, 0.1 to 20 micrometers in size, and are drawn up into the stratosphere where they are transported around the globe on upper winds creating worldwide fallout. They fall to earth weeks to months later. The danger of worldwide fallout is long term. Many of the radioactive materials have very long half lives and settle into the food supply through contamination of fields and waters.

Local fallout is made up of the larger particles, several millimeters in size. They are thrown into the atmosphere and fall to earth in the local area usually within 24 hours. Rain or snow would cause the local fallout to occur sooner. Local fallout poses a significant threat to anyone in the area. Unless evasive or protective measures are taken, a lethal dose through external and internal contamination (through inhalation and ingestion) is likely.[1,2,4]

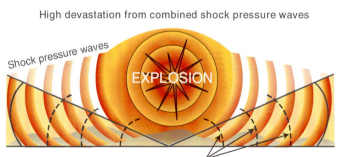

High devastation from combined shock pressure waves

Shock pressure waves

EXPLOSION

Reflected shock waves

FIGURE 10–4. Illustration of Mach Effect of nuclear explosion. The blast wave is reflected off the ground forming an additive effect with the original blast wave. *Courtesy of the Department of Defense.*

ALERT!

Fall out is a great concern from a nuclear explosion. Local fallout occurs when large pieces of radioactive material fall in the local area of the blast over a period of days to weeks. Predominate wind direction, rain, and snow will determine where the fallout will occur and how much will occur in an area. Fallout will cause significant contamination resulting in injury and death to those not protected.

Worldwide fallout is caused by radioactive material vaporized in the immediate area of the explosion that coalesces into very fine particles. These particles are picked up by the winds in the stratosphere and deposited globally. They enter the food chain as they settle in distant fields and waters. The effects of global fallout are long term and may be devastating.

Blast Injuries

Classification

Injuries from explosions are classified into primary, secondary, tertiary, and combined blast injuries. **Primary blast injuries** are those that occur from the overpressure wave caused by the explosion.[5–10] These injuries are increased depending on the size of the explosion, the proximity of the victim to it and to any reflective surfaces, or if victims are in an enclosed space.[5–9,11] The closer the victim is to either the blast or reflective surfaces or in an enclosed space will increase the victim's likelihood of severe injury.

Spallation, implosion, and inertia explain how blast waves cause injury within the body.[5–7,9] **Spallation** occurs when the pressure wave is reflected at the boundary of a denser material causing disruption and explosion of material into the neighboring material. **Implosion** occurs when the pressure wave passes through a liquid that surrounds an air bubble, the air bubble is compressed to a greater degree than it would be by the pressure wave alone. The rapid, explosive decompression of the air bubble causes damage to surrounding tissue, such as damage that occurs in the ear or intestinal tract.[5–9,12] **Inertial effects** are caused by neighboring tissue of differing densities being acted upon by the same blast forces. The lighter of the two objects will move faster than the heavier object causing disruption of the boundaries and organs.[5–10]

Secondary injuries are caused by objects hurled through the air by the blast or dynamic waves caused by the explosion. Explosives may be packed with metal fragments such as nails or ball bearings or the casing of the explosion itself will fragment and be propelled at great force from the explosion. These objects are of a non-aerodynamic shape, which increases the wobble and pitch of the object, making it potentially more damaging to tissue than bullets. Objects near the explosion may be propelled away from the explosion. These objects are propelled farther than the effects of the blast and dynamic waves. This greatly increases the injury and killing distance of explosions.[6–8,10,11]

Tertiary blast injuries occur when the victim is thrown into a solid structure such as a wall and sustains injuries. It is often difficult to differentiate between primary, secondary, and tertiary injuries. Some may be obvious, such as penetrating injuries from fragmentation, which would be secondary injuries. Others from blunt trauma may not be as easily distinguished as secondary, tertiary of possibly primary blast injuries. **Flash and thermal injuries** also are caused by the explosion. Intense heat is generated by explosions and may reach thousands of degrees centigrade. The victim's proximity to the blast or if the blast occurs in an enclosed space will increase the severity of these injuries; those occurring in the open may only cause superficial burns. Burns also may occur from fires ignited from the blast.[7,10,11] The term **combined blast injury** is used to describe injuries from primary, secondary, tertiary, and thermal injuries to a victim.[6–8,10,11]

Primary Blast Injuries

Auditory Blast Injury

The most common blast injury is to auditory system. The auditory system is designed to process sound waves. Blast waves are essentially sound waves of extremely high pressures. The sound from a concert typically is around 0.04 psi.

Overpressures of 1 to 8 psi are needed to cause acute damage to the tympanic membrane.[5,7,10–15]

Damage to the auditory system occurs in the conductive, sensory, or both systems. Rupture to the tympanic membrane is most common, but damage to the ossicular chain also is common. Blast injuries to the inner ear cause transient sensorial hearing loss with tinnitus, vertigo, and balance difficulties, which may be severe and incapacitating in the moments following an explosion. Most victims suffer a degree of damage to both systems.[5,7,10,12]

Treatment consists of removal of any debris in the ear canal and irrigation. Ossicular damage causing vertigo and dizziness has a high incidence of comorbid basilar skull fracture. Examination for cerebral spinal fluid in the ear canal or bruising over the mastoid process (battle signs) would raise the index of suspicion for a basilar skull fracture. Perforations less than a third of the surface of the tympanic membrane should heal spontaneously; large perforations should be referred to a otolaryngologist for further treatment, which may include surgical repair. Sensorial hearing loss may improve with time, but may not improve completely. Residual hearing loss and persistent tinnitus is common.[5,7,10,15] In the past, damage to the auditory system was indicative of impending damage to the lungs, this is no longer found to be true.[5,7,12]

Evidence for Practice

It was commonly thought that tympanic membrane rupture after an explosion was a good indicator for the development of blast lung. In fact, tympanic injury does not necessarily mean that a victim will develop blast lung.

Many internal injuries associated with explosions develop over time and warrant care and observation. Blast lung may develop or will worsen over time and may be exacerbated by treatment if positive-pressure ventilation becomes necessary. Evaluate the victim's pulmonary signs and symptoms over time to evaluate the severity of the injury and effectiveness of treatment.

Blast lung is caused by contusion or barotraumas to the lungs. It is directly proportional to the degree of overpressure exerted on the pulmonary system. As described earlier, damage occurs through the propagation of the blast wave through the varying densities of the lung causing alveolar tears and vascular disruption. The mildest injury takes the form of pleural and subpleural petechiae. Subpleural hemorrhages occur next, particularly near the chest walls and mediastinum where the waves may be reflected. Large parenchymal tears also may occur with stripping of small airway epithelium. Pneumothorax and hemothorax may occur as communication is established between the pleural space and airways. The pneumothorax may become a tension pneumothorax requiring immediate treatment. Traumatic emphysema and alveolo-venous fistula may necessitate intubation and positive-pressure ventilation. This may escalate the chances of pneumothorax in the compromised lung. Gas exchange is impaired at the alveolar level.[10,16] Signs and symptoms include dyspnea, rapid shallow breathing, poor chest wall expansion, cough, hemoptysis, wheezes, and diminished breath sounds.[5–7,10,13,14,17,18]

Victims exposed to overpressures large enough to cause blast lung injuries may also develop air emboli as a complication. Air emboli result from direct communication between the vasculature and the airways. Injuries sustained by the blast wave may cause this or air emboli may be caused by treatment with positive-pressure ventilation. The increased pressure in the airways causes a reversal of the normal pressure gradient between the lungs and the vasculature. Under normal circumstances, the venous pressure is higher than the airway pressure. With positive-pressure ventilation and during the overpressure period from the blast itself (increases in both overpressure and static pressures), the airway pressure is higher than the venous pressure.[5,7] Victims of an explosion in an enclosed area are most at risk for this injury.[5–7,10,11,17,18] These air emboli may be quite small and may affect any vascular bed. Stroke and myocardial infarction are most often the cause of death. Air emboli are often the cause of sudden acute decompensation following intubation and ventilation in a damaged lung. Signs and symptoms may include loss of consciousness, chest pain, peripheral pain and mottling (livido reticularis), or sudden blindness. Arterial blood gases may appear frothy with air bubbles.[5,7,10,13,14,16–18]

Treatment for blast lung is complex with treatment often exacerbating the injuries. The victims are often in shock and have altered levels of consciousness. All victims should be given oxygen via a nonrebreather mask, until more precise methods are possible, allowing highest percentage of oxygen possible. Chest x-ray may be helpful in determining the extent of the injury; however, the fullest extent of the injury may not be evident for hours after the incident. Butterfly infiltrates on x-ray are a sign of blast lung. Acute respiratory distress syndrome (ARDS) may develop. Pulmonary edema may worsen if hypovolemia is treated too aggressively.[5,7,10,13,14,17]

If the victim does need to be intubated and placed on positive-pressure ventilation, steps should be taken to maximize the mean airway pressure while keeping the peak-airway pressure as low as possible. A primary goal is to keep airway pressures lower than vascular pressures thereby decreasing the risk of air emboli while maintaining adequate ventilation and perfusion.[5] Air emboli have formed hours to days after the injury or initiation of positive-pressure ventilation.[10] If it is possible to determine that the lung injury is unilateral and it is possible to determine which lung is injured, it may be possible to intubate only the noninjured lung. Permissive hypercapnia also may be effective in preventing further worsening of barotraumas and the increased risk of air emboli. Positioning the patient may help prevent damage from the air emboli. Trendelenburg positioning may decrease the risk of air emboli entering the cerebral vascular system or keeping the injured lung dependent to the left atrium may prevent the emboli from entering the coronary vasculature. Hyperbaric oxygen therapy (HBOT) is the definitive treatment for systemic air emboli. There are several benefits to HBOT including increased tissue perfusion, decreased intracranial pressure, and decreased reperfusion injury.[5–7,13,14,17,18]

TABLE 10–4   System Injuries From Explosions

SYSTEM	INJURIES
Auditory	Ruptured tympanic membrane
	Inner ear damage
	Hearing loss
Pulmonary	Plural and subpleural petechiae and hemorrhages
	Parenchymal tears
	Hemo/pneumothoracic
	Air emboli
Cardiovascular	Bradycardia
	Hypotension
	Cardiac contusion
Gastrointestinal	Edema
	Delayed hemorrhage and rupture
Central Nervous System	Concussion
	Subdural hematoma
	Diffuse axonal injury

Gastrointestinal Injuries

Gastrointestinal injuries actually occur at lower overpressures than lung injuries but are often overshadowed by the immediacy and life-threatening nature of injury to the lungs. Injuries occur more often to the colon related to larger amounts of air compared to the small bowel. Injuries include edema, hemorrhage, or frank rupture of the bowel. There also may be injury to solid organs such as the spleen and liver through shear forces. Injuries include petechiae, contusions, or lacerations. Victims of underwater explosions who are treading water are at increased risk for gastrointestinal injuries. Severe injuries from rupture of the organs may be delayed as long as 24 to 48 hours after the walls are weakened and scarred by ischemia.[5–7,10–14,19]

Treatment of gastrointestinal blast injury is similar to treatment of any abdominal trauma; nasogastric suction, volume replacement, and surgery as needed. Computed tomography (CT) scans of the abdomen are helpful but may not differentiate between lesions that may potentially rupture versus spontaneous healing.[5,7,13,14,19]

Traumatic Brain Injury

A significant injury associated with the primary blast wave is traumatic brain injury (TBI). The mechanism is not fully understood, but it is thought that the primary blast wave causes concussion, subdural hematoma, and diffuse axonal injury. Diffuse air emboli form causing infarction. Blunt trauma from projectiles or as the victim is thrown into a stationary object also is a source of injury. Symptoms of TBI may include headache, dizziness, irritability, mood changes, fatigue, sleep difficulties, memory impairment, and disordered thinking. Although most people with mild TBI return to full functioning over time, transient consequences such as reduced reaction time and persistent post-concussive symptoms should be expected. Many also develop post-traumatic stress syndrome with lasting effects.[20]

Secondary Blast Injuries

Arguably the majority of injuries caused by an explosion are secondary blast injuries. Casings of explosive devices are designed to fragment into small irregular, yet heavy pieces and are propelled from the blast at great speeds.[10,11] Having a large amount of energy, they cause significant injury to soft tissue. An explosion that causes an overpressure just enough to damage the tympanic membrane is enough to create a blast wind of 70 meters/second or 156 mph. An explosion capable of causing blast lung will generate a blast wind of 400 meters/second or 895 mph. Even though this is not a sustained wind, the initial blast will create missiles of objects near the blast and any objects packed around the explosive device, called shrapnel. In an enclosed space, such as a hallway, the effects are magnified. Wounds created by these fragments are heavily contaminated. They include lacerations and wounds with similar properties as gunshot wounds though often worse related to the odd, non-aerodynamic shape of the fragments. Besides contamination with fragmentation from the explosive device, the wound may have fragments of clothing, dirt, glass, wood, and dust. Dust may "tattoo" the wound creating an area of discoloration.[7,10,13,14,21]

Traumatic amputations are an ominous sign concerning the victim's prognosis. Although not fully understood, it is thought that the primary blast wave shatters the bone at the diaphysis into several fragments; a comminuted fracture. The joint is rarely affected. The dynamic wave and/or shrapnel from the device follows, which rips the soft tissue causing a partial or complete amputation. Reattachment is questionable and depends on the availability of medical facilities, expertise of medical personnel, and manpower. Victim stabilization remains the first priority.[5,7,8,10,13,21–23]

Blast injuries to the eyes are generally related to secondary blast effects. Glass and other foreign bodies may become imbedded, often in both eyes. Foreign bodies will be found both on the surface of the eye and in the interior. Most interior foreign bodies are found in the anterior chamber. They may involve the globe, ocular adnexa, or the orbit. Lid and brow lacerations, sinus and orbital fractures, hyphema, conjunctival hemorrhage, or global rupture may occur. Blindness or severe decrease of visual acuity in one or both eyes is common.[7,10,24]

Treatment of secondary blast wounds needs to be meticulous in debridement, the removal of all foreign material and nonviable tissue. It should be assumed that the wound remains heavily contaminated and therefore not closed acutely. Thoracic and abdominal wounds should be surgically explored. If the victim is hemodynamically unstable, they should be taken immediately to surgery. Soft tissue x-rays for foreign bodies and possible fractures should be considered. Wounds left open to heal should be followed by plastic or general surgery. Tetanus prophylaxis and antibiotics should be administered.[7,10,13,14,21]

Tertiary Blast Injuries

Tertiary injuries are those caused by the victim being thrown into a structure or surface. Although children are more susceptible to being thrown by the blast and dynamic winds, adults also will be affected by winds exceeding hurricane strength. Typical injuries are blunt trauma and sudden deceleration injuries. Treatment is typical of blunt trauma to the thorax and abdomen, including CT scans and surgical interventions. Head and neck injuries are common requiring stabilization in the field with possible surgical intervention in the hospital setting.[7,10,13,14]

Radiation

Radiation injuries from conventional explosives are limited to thermal burns from the fireball of hot gases. Victims must be relatively close to the explosion or in an enclosed area. Radiation injuries from nuclear weapons are the result of both thermal and ionizing radiation. The thermal burns affect victims at greater distances than the ionizing radiation released from the explosion. Local and worldwide fallout increase the effective distance of ionizing radiation.[1,2]

The severity of thermal injuries from explosions is proportional to the victim's proximity to the explosion, the size of the explosion, and the containment of the explosion. In general, thermal injuries from explosions that occur in the open may only be superficial because the thermal energy is allowed to dissipate rapidly. Of course, large explosions or victims close to the explosion may still have significant burns. In a contained area, the thermal energy is not allowed to escape and will cause much more severe thermal injuries.

To understand nuclear radiation injuries, you must first understand radiation. There are four basic types of radiation: alpha particles, beta particles, gamma rays (or x-rays) and neutron. Alpha radiation is two high-energy protons or neutrons. They travel only a few centimeters in the air and only 60 micrometers into the skin. They are not as much of a threat as external radiation as they do not penetrate the outer layer of the skin. They are a threat for internal radiation if inhaled or ingested. Beta radiation is high-speed electrons. They react far less with matter around them than alpha particles, so they penetrate farther into the skin causing ionizing burns. They are particularly dangerous inhaled or ingested.[2]

Gamma radiation and x-rays are the same except for their source. Gamma radiation is released from inside the nucleus of the atom whereas x-rays are emitted from the electron shell. They are photons and have the ability to penetrate deep into tissue. They are highly ionizing. Gamma radiation poses a significant ionizing danger both internally and externally.[2]

Radiation and its potential effect can be measured in different ways. Rads or gray are units used to describe radiation. The term rads is commonly used in the United States whereas gray (Gy) is used internationally; Gy is becoming used more often in the United States. A rad is the deposition of 0.01 joule of energy per kilogram of tissue. It is a onetime dose of radiation.[2]

Rem is a term used to describe and quantify the potential damage caused by radiation. Rem is the term used in the United States whereas sievert (Sv) is the international unit. In a onetime dose, rads and rems will be equal; if the victim is exposed over time to the same radiation, the rems will increase. Ten rads over 10 days would be 100 rems.[2] The conversion factor between Gy and rads or Sv and rems is 100. That is, 1 Gy is equal to 100 rads and 1 Sv is equal to 100 rems.

Four factors should be considered when evaluating the danger of radiation: source, duration, distance, and shielding. The source of the radiation determines the type and amount of radioactivity. Alpha sources may not be as great a concern as gamma sources, depending on the other factors. Distance from the source also greatly affects the amount of radiation the victim receives. When the distance between the victim and the source is doubled, the dose of radiation is four times less. The affect of radiation is also measured over time; by limiting the time of the exposure, the victim's adverse reactions are limited. Lastly, what is between the victim and the source of the radiation is important. Shielding can be anything; however, dense materials generally work better, depending on the type of radiation. The various types of radiation have different penetrating power. Alpha particles may be stopped by a piece of paper; they travel only a few centimeters and will not penetrate broken skin. Beta radiation travels up to 10 feet in the air and can penetrate a few millimeters of skin. Gamma and neutron radiation may travel several hundred feet in the air, can penetrate the whole body, and be damaging to cells. Neutrons also may collide with material, causing it to release gamma radiation. Gamma radiation is shielded by very dense material such as lead, steel, earth, or concrete. Neutrons, because they affect dense material causing them to release gamma radiation, must be shielded by a wax, water, or plastic covering over the dense material.[2]

Working in close proximity to radioactive material can cause significant harm. The amount of damage is a product of the amount of time the person is exposed to and the radioactivity of the material. Measuring the amount of radiation a person is exposed to is extremely important. Those working in close proximity to radioactive material must wear radiation monitoring devices, which should be checked often by trained personnel to ensure that the worker's exposure remains below maximal levels. Long-term health hazards remain throughout the life of the person exposed.

Measuring radiation can be done by portable instruments or personal devices. Portable instruments include Geiger-Müller counters with either an open window or pancake probe, ionizing chamber or neutron meter. The Geiger-Müller counter using an open end wand is used to measure beta and gamma radiation. Adjusting the open end by placing the metal covering over the opening will allow the beta radiation to be shielded and only gamma radiation is measured. By replacing the open end wand with the pancake probe, alpha radiation can be detected. Further, by placing a piece of paper between the probe and the radiation source, alpha particles are shielded and subsequently, beta particles may be shielded with a thin piece of aluminum foil. The aluminum foil will effectively shield both alpha and beta particles, measuring now only gamma radiation. Taking measurements with various shielding material will allow readings for individual types of radiation.[2]

The Geiger-Müller counter works effectively only for low-level doses of radiation. Gamma radiation in particular may saturate the instrument causing it to register a zero when high doses of gamma radiation are present. To measure higher levels of radiation and to measure neutron radiation other instruments are needed. An ionizing chamber is designed to accurately measure higher doses of alpha, beta, and gamma radiation. A neutron meter measures neutron radiation. Neutrons are not ionizing in and of themselves. They interact with other atoms producing gamma radiation. Neutron meters use this interaction to measure the amount of neutron radiation indirectly.[2]

There are several types of personal dosimeters including thermoluminescent (TLD), quartz fiber, neutron, and criticality lockets. TLD dosimeters use impurities added to crystals to absorb radiation. They are then subjected to heat, approximately 200 to 300 degrees centigrade and the light from the release of the energy is measured calculating the dose of radiation. The advantage of this type of dosimeter is that it can measure up to 10 Gy or 1000 rads; however, it requires an equipped laboratory to read the exposure. Quartz fiber dosimeters are essentially ionization chambers with a quartz fiber. As the dose of radiation increases the fiber moves closer to the positive pole. It may measure up to 200mR (radiation measured) per hour. Neutron dosimeters use a type of plastic to track the paths of neutrons and estimate their numbers. Criticality lockets are used when fissionable material is being handled. They measure very high doses of radiation. Lastly, air samplers may be used in conjunction with any of these dosimeters. They sample the air through a filter paper that is then read to determine the dose of radiation.[2]

At the center of a nuclear explosion, a tremendous number of neutrons are released. This radiation has the ability to cause substances around it to become radioactive. Nitrogen in the air, the dirt under the explosion may become radioactive with half-lives of varying lengths. This has the effect of making the area of the explosion radioactive and potentially dangerous for a period of time. Radioactive fallout does not contain such large doses of neutron radiation. It is dangerous to victims exposed, but once the contamination is removed, the victim is not radioactive and poses no threat to those around them. It is imperative that any dust, dirt, or other contaminants be removed quickly from victims. If they are re-contaminated for any reason, the contamination must be removed. It is important to note that any damage done by the radiation is done and will not be increased by the amount of time it may take to perform critical life-saving procedures and care. Critical measures to save the victim's life must come first. If victims die because they are not stabilized, no amount of decontamination would have saved them. The time spent stabilizing them will not increase significantly the injury or concerns caused by the contamination.[1,2]

Personal protective equipment for health-care works varies with the task. For those who are decontaminating grossly contaminated victims, Level C protection, which includes rubber boots, double gloves, Tyvec suits, and powered air-purifying respirators (PAPR) hoods, should be worn. After decontamination, there is little chance of exposure to harmful radiation because the victim does not become radioactive **(see Fig. 10–5).**

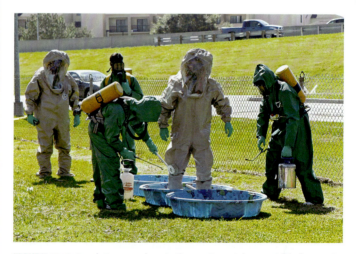

FIGURE 10–5. Level C personal protective equipment is acceptable for use by health-care workers in the hospital or field clinic setting. Level A or B personal protective equipment with self-contained breathing devices are necessary for the field. This is a photograph of responders being scrubbed down after a drill. *Photo by Win Henderson/FEMA.*

Radiation Injuries

Victims may be affected by radiation in several ways. They may be exposed to an external radiation source causing whole body exposure. They may become contaminated after coming externally or internally in contact with radioactive material. Lastly, the radioactive material may become incorporated into a victim's cells, such as when radioactive iodine is taken up by the thyroid gland.[2]

Removing the external gross contamination will minimize beta burns. Beta burns are the result of beta radiation from the contamination. Beta burns do not present in the same manner as thermal burns. There is no immediate reaction. A coppery hue to the skin will develop hours after exposure.[1,2] It is possible to estimate the extent of exposure by the reaction of skin and hair and how quickly beta burns develop. Hair loss or epilation occurs after expose to 3 Gy and takes 2 to 3 weeks to fully develop. Examine the whole body when assessing for hair loss. Beta burns or erythema will develop at differing intervals depending on the dose of radiation. Three Gy will produce erythema in 2 to 3 weeks whereas 6 Gy will produce the effect in 2 to 48 hours. There is no immediate effect on the skin from radiation. Lastly, desquamation occurs at doses above 10 Gy. Dry desquamation occurs as peeling sunburn and is expressed in 2 to 4 weeks. Wet desquamation occurs at doses above 15 to 25 Gy as blistering in about 2 to 8 weeks. At doses of 50 Gy and above, there is a necrosis of the skin that occurs in a much shorter time, days to weeks.[1,2]

Treatment of external contamination is accomplished through the removal of the contaminated material. Clothing should be removed. The victim should be washed gently with soap and water beginning either with specific areas of gross contamination or with the hair. Care should be taken not to contaminate parts of the body not already affected.[1,2]

The affect of internal contamination is dependent on several factors including the type of isotope, its form, and how it entered the body. Isotopes have half-lives that indicate when half of the material is converted into a more stable element or elements. Some radioactive materials have half-lives measured in thousands of years whereas others exist for mere seconds. It takes about 10 half-lives for a material to completely change. The biological half-life is a measure of how long it takes the body to completely remove the isotope. If the form is one that it is not water soluble, the body is able to remove the substance relatively easily. If the substance is in a form easily absorbed by the body, the effect will be more severe. The effective half-life then is a calculation of the biological half-life times the physical half-life divided by the sum of the biological and physical half-lives.[1,2] The normal route of internal contamination is through the lungs or GI tract (mostly the lungs); therefore, steps can be taken to monitor and minimize the effects. Feces should be collected and monitored. The victim should be encouraged to cough vigorously and often and asked to expel or swallow the sputum. Lastly, broncholevage may be used to flush the lungs of radioactive material.[1,2]

Acute Radiation Syndrome

Acute radiation syndrome (ARS) may be defined as a range of injuries caused to body systems that cause illness or death. Radiation rarely kills cells outright; however, it does produce cell death. Cell death is defined as the cells inability to reproduce. As with any exposure, the lethal dose of radiation is expressed as the lethal dose required to kill 50% of those exposed. Creatures with smaller masses require larger doses to be lethal. Time to kill is also a factor because the effects of radiation are not immediate. Originally measured in 30 days, the term $LD_{50/30}$ was used. Human effects may take as long as 60 days so the term $LD_{50/60}$ was used. In general, the term LD_{50} is being used to indicate the dose required to kill 50% of those exposed. Exposure must occur in a high enough dose, very rapidly, and be penetrating radiation. It does not matter if the radiation comes from a terrorist, medical, or industrial source.[1,2]

ARS presents in four phases: prodromal, latent, illness, and outcome. It affects the pulmonary, hematopoietic, gastrointestinal (GI), and central nervous systems (CNS). Each system is affected by differing doses; the hematopoietic system at 2 to 8 Gy, the GI system is affected at 8 to 30 Gy[1,2] **(see Table 10–5).**

The Prodromal Phase

After radiation exposure, the victim will first present with a specific set of symptoms, usually nausea, vomiting, diarrhea, anorexia, and possibly a headache and rise in core temperature.

TABLE 10–5   The Effects of Radiation by Body System

BODY SYSTEM	DOSE OF RADIATION	EFFECT	TIME WITHIN EFFECT OCCURS
Skin	3 Gy	Hair loss and erythema	2–3 weeks
	6 Gy	Hair loss and erythema	2–48 hours
	10 Gy	Dry desquamation	2–4 weeks
	15–25 Gy	Wet desquamation	2–8 weeks
	50 Gy	Necrosis	Few days

Continued

TABLE 10-5 The Effects of Radiation by Body System—cont'd

BODY SYSTEM	DOSE OF RADIATION	EFFECT	TIME WITHIN EFFECT OCCURS
Gastrointestinal	1–2 Gy	Vomiting in a few victims	2–8 hours
	2–4 Gy	Vomiting in most victims	2 hours
	4–8 Gy	Vomiting in all victims	<1 hour
	>8 Gy	Severe vomiting	1–2 weeks
	18–30 Gy	Fatal	
Hematopoietic • Andrew's lymphocyte prognosis	2–8 Gy	Lethal	60 days
	Normal	1500–3000 lymphocytes	
	Moderate	1000–1500 lymphocytes	
	Severe	500–1000 lymphocytes	
	Very severe	100–500 lymphocytes	
	Lethal	<100 lymphocytes	
		measured after 2 days	
Central nervous and cardiovascular system	30 Gy	Lethal due to microvascular damage leading to stroke, cerebral edema, myocardial infarction, failure and death	48 hours

The time from exposure to onset of these symptoms may be a good determinate of how high the dose of radiation was. Vomiting will develop in some of the victims at an exposure of 1 to 2 Gy; 2 to 4 Gy will cause vomiting in most victims in 2 to 8 hours. Four to 8 Gy will cause vomiting in 2 hours, and at doses greater than 8 Gy, vomiting will be severe, starting within the hour.[1,2]

It is important to note that in most radiological incidents, there will be victims actually exposed and those who believe they were. Both will present for care. Because radiation is invisible to the naked eye and its effects are delayed, there is no immediate way to determine who is actually exposed, unless they were wearing a dosimeter. By following the effects on the GI system and the hematopoietic system, specifically the white blood cell count (WBC), it can be determined who was exposed. Vomiting may indicate exposure. Those definitely exposed will show a marked decrease in WBCs in a matter of days, whereas those not exposed will show no change.[1,2]

The Latent Phase

The latent phase follows and the victim feels better. This phase lasts about 2 to 4 weeks though may be shorter with higher doses of radiation. The victim may feel better; however, the systems of the body dependent on fast-growing cells have shut down. Decreased WBCs will cause the victim to begin to develop infections. Anemia will develop. Prophylactic treatment with antibiotics, antifungals and antivirals, and blood and platelet transfusions may be necessary.[1,2]

The Illness Phase

The illness phase follows when damage to specific organ systems begin to be evident. Pulmonary pneumonitis and fibrosis begins to develop. Bone marrow failure causes pancytopenia. The small intestines begin to desquamate, losing their lining. They leak bacteria into the abdomen and fail to function. Veno-occlusive liver disease will develop. Finally, the cardiovascular and CNS systems begin to fail.[1,2]

Definitive Outcome Phase

Within the definitive outcome phase, the victim will either begin to respond to treatment and get better, get better without treatment, as in the case of lower doses of radiation, or die. Recovery may take weeks, months, or the remainder of the victim's life. Specific systems will fail at specific doses of radiation over specific periods of time. The hematopoietic system will receive a lethal dose of 2 to 8 Gy and cause death in 60 days, the GI system lethal dose is 18 to 30 Gy and is fatal in 1 to 2 weeks, and the cardiovascular or central nervous system's lethal dose is 30 Gy and death occurs in 48 hours. Changes occur in the microvascular system of the CNS causing failure. Cerebral edema and increased intracranial pressure develops and is usually fatal.[1,2]

The Andrew's lymphocyte prognosis nomogram may give some indication of victim prognosis. It measures absolute lymphocytes over a 2-day period. Lymphocytes are very susceptible to radiation and will drop precipitously. The normal range of lymphocytes is about 1500 to 3000 absolute lymphocytes. Over 2 days, if the number of absolute lymphocytes drop to between 1000 and 1500 there has been a moderate exposure. A drop to 500 to 1000 indicates a severe exposure, and a drop to 100 to 500 a very severe exposure. Below 100 is lethal[1,2] (see Table 10–5).

Treatment is complex and may not be successful. Complete blood counts (CBCs) should be obtained and repeated every 4 to 6 hours. A sample of blood should be sent for analysis for radioactive sodium. Neutron radiation would produce radioactive sodium in the blood, so this is a good indication of the victim's exposure to neutron radiation. Genetic testing (cytogenetic) of the blood should be carried out. Blood typing should be carried out for the eventual probable need of blood and platelet transfusions. Fecal and urine samples should be analyzed along with nasal swabs to test for internal contamination. The nares trap approximately 5% of the radiation and hold it for about 1.5 hours. Victims with GI, cardiovascular, or central nervous system involvement generally have a very poor prognosis.[1,2]

Summary

Explosives are by far the weapon of choice for terrorist and of the various types, convention explosives used in the form of IEDs (improvised explosive devices) are the most common today. Injuries occur from the heat and debris thrown out from the blast and from the pressure wave. These effects may be magnified by the reflection of this wave off solid objects such as the ground or structures. Nuclear explosions cause far more extensive damage and injury because of the magnitude of the explosion and the effects of radiation. Injuries from explosions range from relatively minor damage to the tympanic membrane to severe fatal injuries to major organ systems. Radiation injuries range from mild nausea and fatigue to death related to the dose of radiation the victim is exposed to. Decontamination of the victim of radiation is essential but not as essential as treating life-threatening injuries. Concerning radiation, it is far more important to have a live victim who remains contaminated for a short period of time than a dead clean victim. Dirty bombs may spread contaminated material over a wide area; however, most of the injuries will occur from the blast itself, not the radiation. In spite of the small chance of radiation injuries, these weapons may cause a significant amount of panic from the general public and decontaminating the affected area may be very difficult (see Fig. 10–6).

Health-care providers including nurses should be prepared to treat a wide variety of injuries related to the use of both conventional and nuclear explosives. Severe trauma from a variety of causes, thermal burns, and possibly radiation injuries will require the health-care community to work as a team for the victim beginning at the scene and continuing through recovery and rehabilitation. In cases of nuclear explosions and conventional explosions (because of the threat of a dirty bomb) there may also be a large number of worried well victims who believe they have been contaminated and desperately need to be decontaminated. The disaster plan of any health-care institution must include steps to care for these large numbers of victims and provide for the security of providers and victims alike.

Nursing should anticipate the care and treatment of these victims. Registered nurses should be an integral part of the health-care team and advanced practice nurses, along with physicians directing care through all of the phases of patient care. This requires knowledge and skill dependent on both education and experience.

Lastly, this is an area where research is essential. Many life-saving procedures have been developed through caring for victims of war and wounded warriors. Many more are being developed as they are cared for through recovery and rehabilitation. Nursing research can and is playing a significant role in the care of these injured throughout these phases.

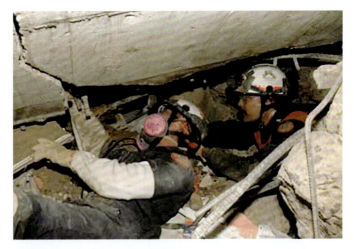

FIGURE 10–6. Oklahoma City, Oklahoma, April 26, 1995. Task Force members maneuver through a crawl space in collapsed Alfred P. Murrah Federal Building in Oklahoma City. Most large terrorist or industrial explosions will result in large numbers of victims presenting to the hospital for treatment. *FEMA News Photo.*

REFERENCES

1. Hogan DE, Burnstein JL, eds. *Disaster Medicine*. Philadelphia, PA: Lippincott Williams & Wilkins, 2002, 432.

2. Keyes DC, ed. *Medical Response to Terrorism*. Philadelphia, PA: Lippincott Williams & Wilkins; 2005, 449.

3. Department of the Navy. Introduction to Naval Weapons Engineering. 1998.

4. Department of Defense. NUCLEAR WEAPONS EFFECTS TECHNOLOGY, M.C.T.L. (MCTL), Editor. 2008.

5. Ritenour AE, Baskin TW. Primary blast injury: update on diagnosis and treatment. *Critical Care Medicine*. 2008;36(7 Suppl):S311–S317.

6. Gruss E. A correction for primary blast injury criteria. *Journal of Trauma*. 2006;60(6):1284–1289.

7. Wightman JM, Gladish SL. Explosions and blast injuries. *Annals of Emergency Medicine*. 2001;37(6):664–678.

8. Eastridge BJ. Things that go boom: injuries from explosives. *Journal of Trauma*. 2007;62(6 Suppl):S38.

9. Langworthy MJ, Sabra J, Gould M. Terrorism and blast phenomena: lessons learned from the attack on the USS Cole (DDG67). *Clinical Orthopaedics and Related Research*. 2004;(422):82–87.

10. Crabtree J. Terrorist homicide bombings: a primer for preparation. *Journal of Burn Care and Research*. 2006;27(5):576–588.

11. Leibovici D, Gofrit ON, Stein M, et al. Blast injuries: bus versus open-air bombings—a comparative study of injuries in survivors of open-air versus confined-space explosions. *Journal of Trauma*. 1996;41(6):1030–1035.

12. Leibovici D, Gofrit ON, Shapira SC. Eardrum perforation in explosion survivors: is it a marker of pulmonary blast injury? *Annals of Emergency Medicine*. 1999;34(2):168–172.

13. Almogy G, Belzberg H, Mintz Y, et al. Suicide bombing attacks: update and modifications to the protocol. [see comment]. *Annals of Surgery*. 2004;239(3):295–303.

14. Almogy G, Luria T, Richter E, et al. Can external signs of trauma guide management?: lessons learned from suicide bombing attacks in Israel. *Archives of Surgery*. 2005;140(4):390–393.

15. Kozuka M, Nakashima T, Fukuta S, Yanagita N. Inner ear disorders due to pressure change. *Clinical Otolaryngology and Allied Sciences*. 1997;22(2):106–110.

16. Irwin RJ, Lerner MR, Bealer JF, Brackett DJ, Tuggle DW. Cardiopulmonary physiology of primary blast injury. *Journal of Trauma*. 1997;43(4):650–655.

17. Sorkine P, Szold O, Kluger Y, et al. Permissive hypercapnia ventilation in patients with severe pulmonary blast injury. *Journal of Trauma*. 1998;45(1):35–38.

18. Bass CR, Rafaels KA, Salzar S. Pulmonary injury risk assessment for short-duration blasts. *Journal of Trauma*. 2008;65(3):604–615.

19. Paran H, Neufeld D, Shwartz I, et al. Perforation of the terminal ileum induced by blast injury: delayed diagnosis or delayed perforation? *Journal of Trauma*. 1996;40(3):472–475.

20. Martin EM, Lu WC, Helmich K, French L, Warden DL. Traumatic brain injuries sustained in the Afghanistan and Iraq wars. *American Journal of Nursing*. 2008;108(4):40–47; quiz 47–48.

21. Langworthy, MJ, Smith JM, Gould M. Treatment of the mangled lower extremity after a terrorist blast injury. *Clinical Orthopaedics and Related Research*. 2004;(422):88–96.

22. Frykberg ER. Medical management of disasters and mass casualties from terrorist bombings: How can we cope? *Journal of Trauma*. 2002;53(2):201–212.

23. Frykberg ER, Tepas JJ 3rd. Terrorist bombings. Lessons learned from Belfast to Beirut. *Annals of Surgery*. 1988;208(5):569–576.

24. Muzaffar W, Khan MD, Akbar KM, et al. Mine blast injuries: ocular and social aspects. *British Journal of Ophthalmology*. 2000;84(6):626–630.

References

11

This section of the book deals with national, state, and local references that may provide education, information, and other help in preparing for or dealing with an emergency or disaster. The national section contains Web sites, phone numbers, and other information. The state and local sections have headings with fill-in lines where you can add the appropriate contact information. List phone numbers and/or Web pages. Be sure to add emergency numbers and non-emergency numbers. Check the numbers and Web sites regularly. They change. If you need them, you do not want to find out that their number changed and you do not have the new one.

National

Below you will find a short list of Web sites that provide information, education, and help when responding to or planning for a disaster.

http://www.dhs.gov/xprepresp/
Department of Homeland Security Web site—Preparedness and Response. This site contains a wealth of information, links, and publications concerning disaster preparation and response.
Links available include:

- Activities & Programs
- Committees & Working Groups
- Laws & Regulations
- Grants
- Training & Technical Assistance

- Publications
- Local Resources

The home site provides links for:

- Citizens
- First Responders
- Business
- Government
- Job Seekers

Other tabs include research, prevention and protection, information sharing, and more.

http://emergency.cdc.gov/
The Center for Disease Control and Prevention Web site provides information concerning bioterrorism, chemical emergencies, mass casualty incidents, radiation, and a multitude of other illnesses and concerns. Training and exercises can be accessed. Contact phone number is provided.

http://www.nnepi.org/
This is a Homeland Security site for nursing. It is the National Nurse Emergency Preparedness Initiative. The site contains links for training programs and information specifically designed for hospital, school public health, and other nursing groups.

http://www.fbi.gov/
The Federal Bureau of Investigation Web site provides information concerning reporting terrorist networks and activities. Local phone numbers are listed along with links for resources, education, and crime information.

http://training.fema.gov/IS/
Federal Emergency Management Agency (FEMA) Independent Study Web site. This Web site has several courses that range from personal preparedness to the Incident Command System and the National Incident Management System and

the National Response plan. The courses are updated and certificates are offered for the completion of each course. A multiple-choice test is given at the end of each course over the Internet. There is no cost.

http://www.citizencorps.gov/cert/
The Community Emergency Response Team (CERT) Program educates people about disaster preparedness for hazards that may impact their area and trains them in basic disaster response skills, such as fire safety, light search and rescue, team organization, and disaster medical operations. Using the training learned in the classroom and during exercises, CERT members can assist others in their neighborhood or workplace following an event when professional responders are not immediately available to help. CERT members also are encouraged to support emergency response agencies by taking a more active role in emergency preparedness projects in their community. (Taken from the CERT Web site.)

https://hseep.dhs.gov/pages/1001_HSEEP7.aspx
The Homeland Security Exercise and Evaluation Program (HSEEP) is a capabilities and performance-based exercise program that provides a standardized methodology and terminology for exercise design, development, conduct, evaluation, and improvement planning.

The Homeland Security Exercise and Evaluation Program (HSEEP) constitutes a national standard for all exercises. Through exercises, the National Exercise Program supports organizations to achieve objective assessments of their capabilities so that strengths and areas for improvement are identified, corrected, and shared as appropriate prior to a real incident. To learn more about the HSEEP program, click on the About HSEEP tab listed above.

The HSEEP is maintained by the Federal Emergency Management Agency's National Preparedness Directorate, Department of Homeland Security. (Taken from the HSEEP Web site.)

http://www.nfaonline.dhs.gov/

U.S. Fire Administration/FEMA Web site with online training available.

http://www.dhs.gov/xabout/history/gc_1193938363680.shtm

The National Strategy for Homeland Security guides, organizes, and unifies our nation's homeland security efforts. Homeland security is a responsibility shared across our entire nation, and the strategy provides a common framework for the following four goals:

- Prevent and disrupt terrorist attacks.
- Protect the American people, our critical infrastructure, and key resources.
- Respond to and recover from incidents that do occur.
- Continue to strengthen the foundation to ensure our long-term success.

This updated Strategy, which builds directly from the first National Strategy for Homeland Security issued in July 2002, reflects our increased understanding of the terrorist threats confronting the United States today, incorporates lessons learned from exercises and real-world catastrophes—including Hurricane Katrina—and proposes new initiatives and approaches that will enable the Nation to achieve our homeland security objectives.

This site contains PDF documents and other information. (Taken from the National Strategy for Homeland Security Web site.)

http://www.dhs.gov/xprepresp/committees/editorial_0566.shtm

The National Response Framework (NRF) presents the guiding principles that enable all response partners to prepare for and provide a unified national response to disasters and emergencies. It establishes a comprehensive, national, all-hazards approach to domestic incident response. The

National Response Plan was replaced by the National Response Framework effective March 22, 2008.

The National Response Framework defines the principles, roles, and structures that organize how we respond as a nation. The National Response Framework:

- Describes how communities, tribes, states, the federal government, private-sectors, and nongovernmental partners work together to coordinate national response.
- Describes specific authorities and best practices for managing incidents.
- Builds upon the National Incident Management System (NIMS), which provides a consistent template for managing incidents.

Information on the National Response Framework including Documents, Annexes, References and Briefings/Trainings can be accessed from the NRF Resource Center.

State

State or Regional Public Health

_____

_____

_____

Regional Poison Control

_____

_____

_____

Regional Trauma Center

_____

_____

_____

Regional Burn Center

_____

_____

_____

State or Regional Emergency Preparedness Agency

_____

_____

_____

State Police

_____

_____

_____

State Emergency Planning and Response

_____

_____

_____

School Preparedness State Councils

_____

_____

_____

State Advisory Councils on Preparedness

_____

_____

_____

State Child Preparedness Agency

_____

_____

_____

Local

Local Police Department

_____

_____

_____

Local Sheriff Department

_____

_____

_____

EMS/Fire/Emergency

_____

_____

_____

Fire Department non-emergency

_____

_____

_____

Health Department

_____

_____

_____

Water and Sanitation Department

_____

_____

_____

Local Emergency Planning

_____

_____

_____

Local Emergency Management Office

_____

_____

_____

Other notes and information.

_____

_____

_____

_____

_____

_____

_____

_____

_____

_____

_____

_____

_____

_____

_____

_____

Index